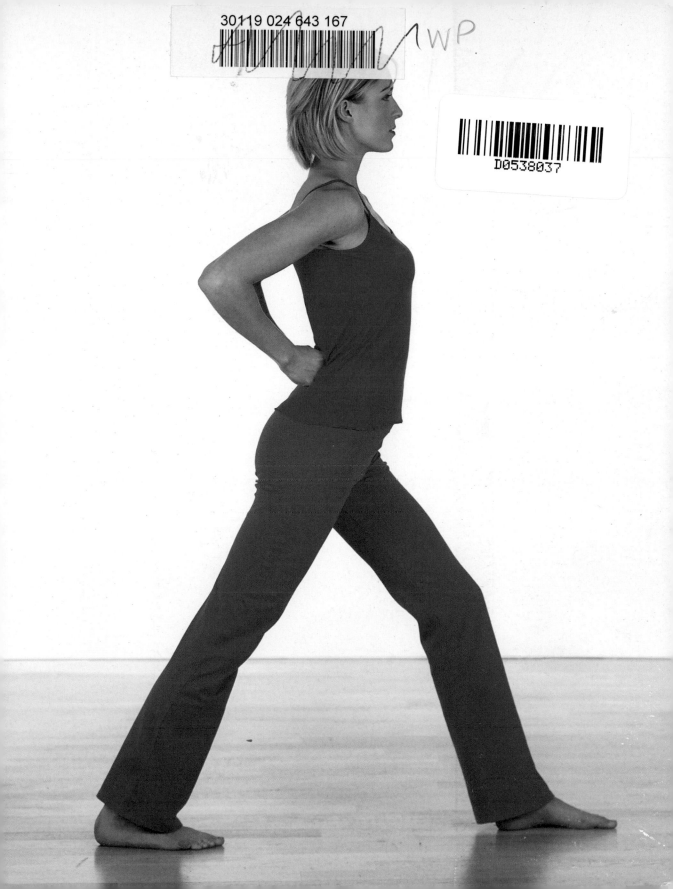

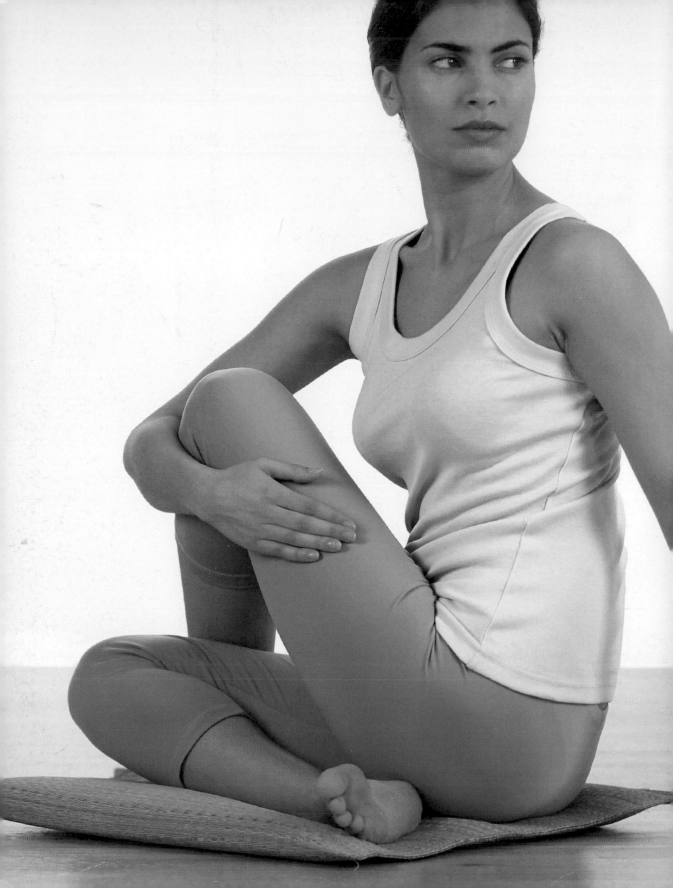

SUZANNE MARTIN PT, DPT

stretching

The stress-free way to stay supple,
keep fit, and exercise safely

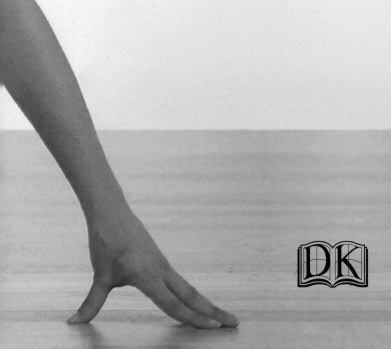

DK

LONDON, NEW YORK, MELBOURNE, MUNICH, DELHI

For Jeanne and J.B. Clements

Project Editor **Nasim Mawji**
Project Art Editor **Miranda Harvey**
Managing Editors **Stephanie Farrow, Penny Warren**
Managing Art Editor **Marianne Markham**
Publishing Manager **Gillian Roberts**
Art Director **Carole Ash**
Publishing Director **Mary-Clare Jerram**
DTP Designer **Sonia Charbonnier**
Production Controller **Elizabeth Warman**
Photographer **Russell Sadur**

First published in Great Britain in 2005
by Dorling Kindersley Limited
80 Strand, London WC2R 0RL
Penguin Group (UK)

2 4 6 8 10 9 7 5 3 1

Always consult your doctor before starting a fitness
programme if you have any health concerns.

A CIP catalogue record for this book is available
from The British Library

ISBN 1 4053 0350 6

Colour reproduction by Colourscan, Singapore
Printed and bound by Tien Wah Press, Singapore

Discover more at
www.dk.com

CONTENTS

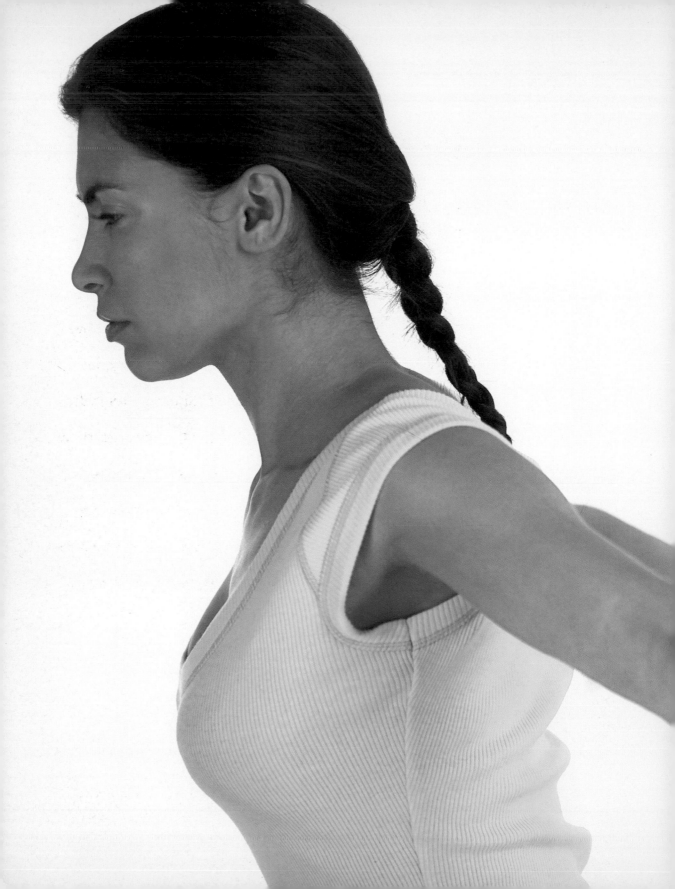

WHAT IS STRETCHING?

Welcome to one of life's great pleasures. Stretching is for everyone, young and old, from all walks of life. You don't have to be a contortionist, professional athlete, or even in good shape to experience its joys and benefits. Stretching can help you to feel better and even to look better. This book will show you how to make it part of your lifestyle. You'll learn about the many ways that stretching can enhance your day-to-day activities, whether by improving your performance at sports, or just by making reaching up to a high shelf that little bit easier.

DEFINING STRETCHING

In this book I will show you how stretching can truly transform your life. It is a simple and instantly gratifying form of physical release that can energize you in the morning or relax you at night. It can enhance your enjoyment of sports or ease a stiff neck after a long telephone call. I believe that stretching is as crucial to the proper functioning of the body as oxygen.

An essential component of fitness

Along with cardiovascular exercise (which raises your heart rate) and resistance training (lifting weights), stretching is an essential component of a complete fitness regime, yet it is often the most neglected. People either perceive it as too easy and, as a result, unnecessary, or too difficult, believing that only the very flexible actually benefit from stretching.

In fact, regular, controlled stretching improves and maintains flexibility and mobility, corrects bad posture, reduces the risk of injury, relieves pain, and even helps counteract the effects of ageing. In addition, it relaxes the body, helps reduce stress levels, and can help to boost self-esteem. Everyone, regardless of age or fitness level, can benefit from stretching. By making it an integral part of your lifestyle, you will reap its many benefits.

Is it like yoga?

Many people think of yoga or Pilates when they think of stretching. Yoga's original goal was to increase flexibility for the positions of meditation. Pilates is often called moving yoga, but the main goals are torso strength and control. Both yoga and Pilates follow a strict form and require expert instruction to avoid injury. Stretching is different, in that it is simple. It aims to align the body, improve posture, and encourage better mechanical movement of the joints, which reduces wear and tear on them. Put simply, stretching helps the body to work harmoniously.

Stretching affects more than the 602 muscles of the body. When you stretch muscles, you also mobilize joints, elongate skin, and affect connective tissue, nerves, tendons, and sometimes ligaments.

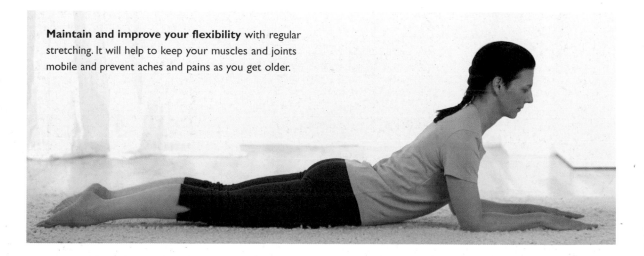

Maintain and improve your flexibility with regular stretching. It will help to keep your muscles and joints mobile and prevent aches and pains as you get older.

The rebalancing effect of stretching

Think of stretching as a way of rebalancing the body. Our muscles come in a variety of shapes and sizes. Arranged around joints, they move in many complex ways. Sometimes making a simple action can involve as many as 19 muscles. If one or more of these muscles is used improperly, you feel it, and not always in the most obvious place. A client may come to me with a painful shoulder, but the cause may be tight chest muscles that pull on the joint and put it under strain. Similarly, there may be a complaint of a sore lower back, but the real culprits may be tight muscles at the backs of the thighs and rigid muscles in the ribcage. It's known as the noisy victim and silent criminal syndrome.

Functional stretching, stretching for daily life, doesn't require special equipment. It can be enjoyed anywhere and at any time. Often the stretches are so subtle that people won't realize what you're doing. When you stretch more dramatically, the pleasure is obvious – you may even notice that people copy you.

Stretching is as essential as breathing in counteracting the wear and tear of everyday life and activity. And the wonderful thing is that beginners stand to benefit just as much as advanced movers – even flexible people need to balance their muscles. Make stretching part of your lifestyle, and you'll make your body a friend for life.

Take pleasure in stretching – enjoy the feeling of release that comes from lengthening and elongating your muscles.

WHY WE MUST STRETCH

Stretching improves flexibility and energizes the body, but it is also important for good posture. Over our lifetimes, the constant downwards pull of gravity and the dehydrating effects of ageing cause us gradually to hunch our shoulders and – more alarmingly – to shrink. Regular stretching can help you achieve an upright and energetic posture and a vital, healthy, and pain-free body.

Our bodies suffer daily fatigue from fighting against the constant downwards pull of gravity. At the same time, ageing has a dehydrating effect, and as we grow older, our bodily tissues become leathery. After years of being right- or left-handed and performing regular activities such as sitting and driving, we start to stiffen into the positions we have assumed through the years. The effect is to leave you sagging, hunched over, and too tired to carry on. However, this doesn't have to be a death sentence. You can counteract the effects of gravity and ageing on the body and achieve your ideal posture with a stretching programme that balances muscular irregularities.

Typical bad posture

Look at the figure on the right. Her stooped posture is typical of the effects of gravity and ageing. She has an overall saggy appearance – as if she is literally being dragged down. A tight neck and face give the impression of being tired and strained – she really looks as if she carries the weight of the world on her shoulders. Her hunched shoulders are the result of tight chest muscles and practically guarantee arm and hand pain over time. The rotator cuff muscles of the shoulder are literally pinched by this forwards position, which often causes pain and discomfort. A tight lower back not only leads to an unsightly protruding abdomen, it compresses the nerves and can lead to sciatica, leg pain, or, worse yet, problems with bathroom and sexual functions. Tight front of hip muscles intensify the forwards sway of

the lower back and often lead to knee problems, the scourge of females as they are already prone to knee problems because of genetically wider hips. In pronounced cases, the forwards sway of the lower back can give an unsightly appearance to the bottom. Tight hamstrings inevitably cause lower back pain. The calves and feet are notoriously tight because we are on them all day. Tight calves can lead to a painful yet preventable injury, Achilles' tendon rupture. Tight feet tend to lead to plantar fasciitis, an uncomfortable heel condition.

Ideal body posture

Now look at the figure on the far right. Notice what a huge difference good posture makes to how you perceive this person: bright, confident, and athletic. Her face is no longer strained because her head is back over the line of her pelvis. Her neck is now swan-like. Once the shoulders are back and the chest is open, the forlorn look is replaced by an open, relaxed one. Her ears now line up over her shoulders. The rotator cuff can move the arm in its socket the way it was intended. The waist is elongated because the lower back is lengthened. Sitting will now be easier. The abdomen is sleek and no longer protrudes. The hips are upright and forwards, which will help her to stand for long periods without feeling tired. The pelvis is positioned more forwards on the feet, enabling more bounce in the step and that "go to it" feeling that gives motivation to take on a new day.

TYPICAL BAD POSTURE

Tight muscles pull the skeleton out of alignment, creating awkward and ungainly posture. Muscle aches and pains are common for this person.

IDEAL POSTURE

The head aligns over the pelvis, the shoulders are back, and the muscles are balanced, giving a sleek, streamlined appearance.

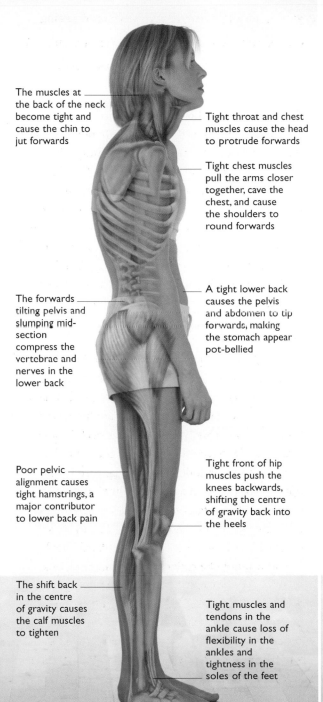

The muscles at the back of the neck become tight and cause the chin to jut forwards

Tight throat and chest muscles cause the head to protrude forwards

Tight chest muscles pull the arms closer together, cave the chest, and cause the shoulders to round forwards

The forwards tilting pelvis and slumping mid-section compress the vertebrae and nerves in the lower back

A tight lower back causes the pelvis and abdomen to tip forwards, making the stomach appear pot-bellied

Poor pelvic alignment causes tight hamstrings, a major contributor to lower back pain

Tight front of hip muscles push the knees backwards, shifting the centre of gravity back into the heels

The shift back in the centre of gravity causes the calf muscles to tighten

Tight muscles and tendons in the ankle cause loss of flexibility in the ankles and tightness in the soles of the feet

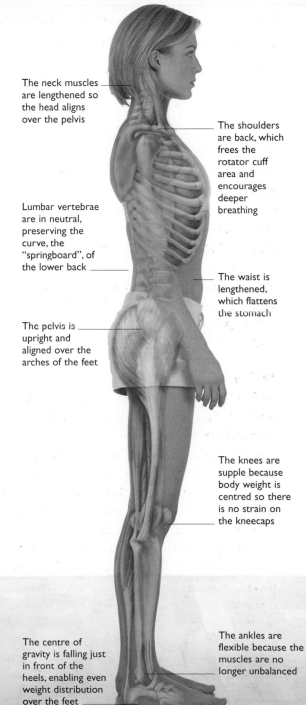

The neck muscles are lengthened so the head aligns over the pelvis

The shoulders are back, which frees the rotator cuff area and encourages deeper breathing

Lumbar vertebrae are in neutral, preserving the curve, the "springboard", of the lower back

The waist is lengthened, which flattens the stomach

The pelvis is upright and aligned over the arches of the feet

The knees are supple because body weight is centred so there is no strain on the kneecaps

The centre of gravity is falling just in front of the heels, enabling even weight distribution over the feet

The ankles are flexible because the muscles are no longer unbalanced

What happens when you stretch?

Strong muscles, tendons, bones, and ligaments are essential to maintain a healthy, vital body that will serve you well for your entire life. As soon as you go into a stretch you immediately begin to feel the pull of your muscles upon your bones. Tendons connect muscles to bones, and the pull of stretching can help the tendons to "plump up", helping to prevent the injuries that occur all too often when exercising or just carrying out everyday activities.

Ligaments connect bone to bone and hold the skeleton together. The aim when stretching correctly is to elongate the muscles and tendons while protecting the ligaments – you don't want them to stretch. Each muscle has an optimum length, and this book will show you which ones to stretch and where so that you achieve your ideal posture. Focused and correct stretching helps align the spine and balance the muscle groups that would otherwise become shortened by gravity over time.

As we age and our bodies slowly dehydrate, stretching is even more important. In the same way that this slow process of dehydration causes wrinkles on the exterior, it also affects the body tissues inside our skin. Not only do our muscles, tendons, and ligaments dry out and tighten, they become leathery. Over time this causes the body to stiffen, gradually giving a stooped appearance, but it also begins to block the healthy circulation of nutrients around the body.

> ### THE BENEFITS OF STRETCHING
>
> Listed below are just some of the many physical and mental benefits that stretching has to offer:
>
> - helps balance muscle lengths, which aligns the body, improving and correcting posture
> - improves flexibility and mobility so that sitting, walking, and standing become easier
> - helps counteract the effects of ageing by promoting circulation of nutrients and water throughout the body
> - reduces risk of injury by improving flexibility and balance
> - promotes relaxation and reduces stress
> - energizes body, mind, and spirit.

Stretching affects not only our muscle system, but also our neurological system, which includes the operation of the brain. When you stretch, you lengthen some areas while relaxing others. The brain in turn regulates automatic functions such as heart rate and blood pressure. It secretes hormones, which act as chemical messengers to help insulin control, metabolism, mood, and emotion.

Besides the internal physiological benefits come the day-to-day benefits of being flexible enough to sit without experiencing back and shoulder pain. Simple actions such as bending down to small

Knee joint
Joint mobility is improved through regular stretching of the muscles around a joint

A stretch may target a muscle, or group of muscles, but its benefits will be felt throughout the body, and even on a mental level.

children or reaching up to a high shelf all become easier. Walking and stair climbing become more efficient so that you use less energy and, as a result, feel less tired during the day.

Along with the physical benefits come untold emotional and mental ones. Stretching is the original mind-body activity. It slows you down so that your heart and mind can come together to achieve an inner calmness. Many a time a simple stretch can put a problem in perspective, and so a better solution can be found to life's many dilemmas.

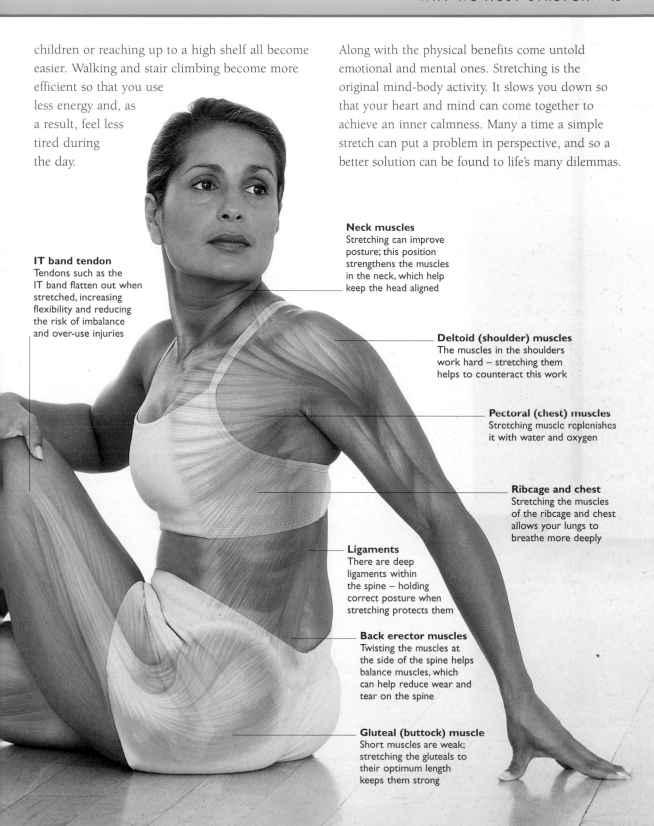

IT band tendon
Tendons such as the IT band flatten out when stretched, increasing flexibility and reducing the risk of imbalance and over-use injuries

Neck muscles
Stretching can improve posture; this position strengthens the muscles in the neck, which help keep the head aligned

Deltoid (shoulder) muscles
The muscles in the shoulders work hard – stretching them helps to counteract this work

Pectoral (chest) muscles
Stretching muscle replenishes it with water and oxygen

Ribcage and chest
Stretching the muscles of the ribcage and chest allows your lungs to breathe more deeply

Ligaments
There are deep ligaments within the spine – holding correct posture when stretching protects them

Back erector muscles
Twisting the muscles at the side of the spine helps balance muscles, which can help reduce wear and tear on the spine

Gluteal (buttock) muscle
Short muscles are weak; stretching the gluteals to their optimum length keeps them strong

HOW TO STRETCH

Stretching is exercise made simple. It is easy to perform, and requires minimum exertion to feel fantastic benefits. From the very beginning, the sensation of breathing into a stretch will make you feel better. You'll notice that little aches and pains disappear, and you'll be drawn in to want more. Here I outline some simple guidelines to ensure sensible, effective, and pleasurable stretching.

Form and focus

Attention to form helps ensure that you get the most out of a stretch. Most of the stretches in this book are elongation stretches, where you hold one part of the body and stretch the other against it. Do your best to get into the positions demonstrated. If you can't replicate a stretch exactly, get as close as you can to it. Use the "feel it here" patches as guides to where you feel a stretch when you are performing it correctly. Gently ease into a position, check how it feels, then focus on the muscles being stretched. Never bounce. Be careful not to push yourself too far – respect your body's limitations. Although the positions may feel awkward or unfamiliar at first, there should never be any pain. A good elongation stretch feels as if you are reaching a gentle barrier of tension, then as you slowly ease into the stretch, you should feel that barrier give way. If you hold an elongation stretch too tautly and overstretch, your muscle will actually pull back against you.

This book also features some moving stretches, where you follow a movement pattern. Generally, the movements should always be slow and smooth but as rhythmic as possible. An effective moving stretch feels like a release.

Attention to good form and technique will ensure that you benefit fully from a stretch and don't risk injury. Focus, and work with your body, not against it.

Finally, respect your body type. Some people are more flexible in their ligaments by nature. If you can touch your thumb to your forearm, or if your elbows or knees are naturally hyperextended (they bend back slightly), you are more flexible than the general population. Lanky people tend to be flexible in the joints. If this sounds like you, take care. Try not to push yourself into extreme end-of-range positions. No matter what, if you feel apprehension about a position, your intuition is trying to tell you something. Come out of the stretch and work out how to make the position smaller and more precise.

Breathing

Be sure to breathe deeply and rhythmically throughout a stretch. People tend to hold their breath or forget to breathe when concentrating on or counting out a stretch. Instead of counting, I recommend that you hold a stretch for a number of breath cycles. (A breath cycle is a deep breath in and then out.) Breathing deeply helps you to relax and will actually help you to ease further into a stretch without straining. Even during a moving stretch, it's important to remember to breathe.

Stabilizing

One key element in elongation stretching is the need for a stabilizing anchor – something stable that you can stretch away from in order to lengthen a particular body part. In standing positions, gently squeezing the buttocks "anchors" the pelvis and prevents it from twisting or tilting. Lifting the groin or pelvic floor adds to the effect. (Similar to Kegel exercises, this should feel as if an elevator is going up the inside of the body from the bottom of the pelvis.) Pulling your navel into the spine refers to abdominal and back control. Contracting your back and abdominal muscles stabilizes the spine and ensures that you protect it and prevent any ligament damage than can result from overstretching a joint.

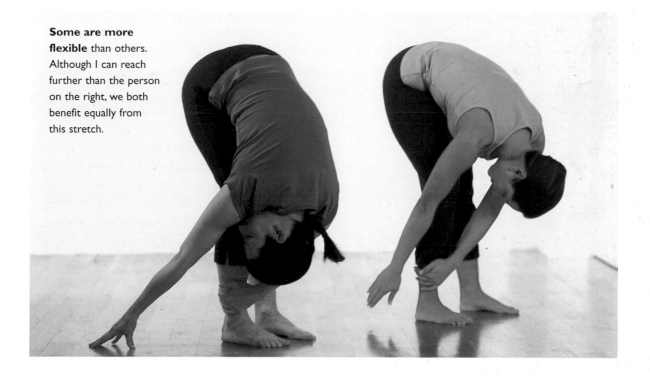

Some are more flexible than others. Although I can reach further than the person on the right, we both benefit equally from this stretch.

GETTING STARTED

Stretching is for people of all ages and abilities. If you are new to it, start gradually – devote just a few minutes a day to it and you'll soon feel the benefits. Don't compare yourself to others; use stretching to get to know your own body better. Follow these simple suggestions to help you get started – and to enjoy stretching for the rest of your life!

How to use this book

Getting started is easy. I recommend that everyone begin with the simple Flexibility Test (*see pp.18–19*). This helps you to identify how flexible you are naturally, but it also helps you to pinpoint tight areas that may need more attention.

If you're a beginner, a good place to start is the 21-day Posture Programme (*see pp.52–65*). The main goal is to make stretching a lifestyle and a part of your daily routine. The programme requires only 15 minutes a day for three weeks and yet it can produce truly remarkable results. It's a fantastic advertisement for the benefits of regular stretching.

Alternatively, whether you are a beginner or a more practised stretcher, consult the Head-to-Toe Catalogue of Stretches (*see pp.20–51*) to target particular areas of the body that need work. There are numerous stretches for different sports, activities, and times of life contained within these pages. There are also therapeutic stretches to help you to deal with typical problem areas such as the neck and shoulders and lower back. The beauty of this book is that you have many stretches from which to pick and choose, creating hundreds of new variations of sequences.

When to stretch

Ideally, you should aim to stretch daily, whether you're a beginner or a regular stretcher. You don't have to wait between days as with weight training. If you plan to stretch every day, choose a convenient time and make it part of your routine. Find the time or times that work best in your schedule, whether early in the morning or last thing at night. Try to integrate stretching into your day whenever

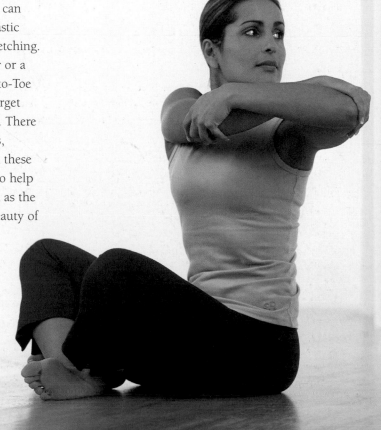

Notice how you feel when you stretch. How does your body respond? Can you twist as far to the right as you can to the left?

possible. During long periods at the computer, get into the habit of taking regular stretching breaks; take five minutes to perform a short routine after a flight or a long drive.

One common misconception is that you should stretch to warm up before sports. A pre-sport warm-up should consist mainly of swinging, rhythmic movements that help to limber you up. The idea is to increase circulation and body heat, not lengthen the muscles. Over-stretching before sports can actually decrease strength and reaction times.

What to wear

You don't need special clothing for stretching, especially if you are gardening, travelling, or playing a sport. Wear anything comfortable that won't make you feel too hot or cold. Any athletic wear or loose clothing will do, so will leggings and a tee shirt. Wear whatever suits your lifestyle, as long as the clothes don't restrict your movements.

Medical considerations

Respect your body's limitations: stretch judiciously. If you have specific body problems, such as lower back and neck complaints or old shoulder injuries, consult your doctor and confirm that these stretches are safe for you to perform.

A word about pregnancy

Gentle stretching is generally safe and beneficial during pregnancy and after the birth. To be absolutely certain of safety, check with your doctor before you begin stretching, especially if you are new to it. The body produces a hormone called relaxin during pregnancy and up to about three months after childbirth (and the same applies for miscarriages). Relaxin relaxes the muscles and tendons in preparation for childbirth, but it may also put you at risk of stretching beyond your normal range. Do take care – don't push yourself. Use any suggested props to ensure your comfort (*see* Props *below*).

PROPS

For some stretches, I might suggest that you use a prop, either to make a position more comfortable (which will help you to relax and stretch more effectively), or to help you to maintain good form. In some cases, a prop such as a tennis ball can help you to target specific tight muscles. These props are all items that you should have around the home.

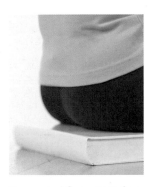

For seated floor stretches, try sitting on a phone book to help straighten your back and relieve pressure on the sides of the feet.

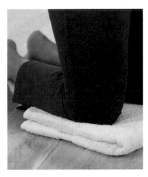

For kneeling stretches, try placing a folded towel under the knees to cushion them and help make the position more comfortable.

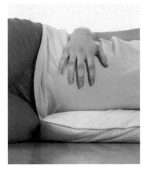

For pregnancy stretches that involve lying on your side, place a pillow or cushion under your waist for support.

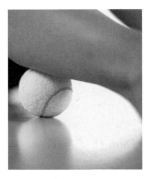

In some cases, applying pressure with a tennis ball can help to focus a stretch – for example, in the calves, back, or soles of feet.

HOW FLEXIBLE AM I?

Flexibility differs from one person to the next. Even the most pliable people have areas of the body that need work – they tend to stretch only the areas and in the directions in which they are most flexible. Use this series of tests to help isolate less flexible areas of the body, those that will really benefit noticeably from regular stretching.

Although the tests are demonstrated on one side of the body, be sure to test your flexibility on both sides. Each test provides a guide to measure your degree of flexibility. Notice how you feel in the positions, and compare your side-to-side results. Is your right leg tighter than your left? Is any body part talking to you? Then use the Head-to-Toe Catalogue of Stretches (*see pp.20–51*) to help you target specific areas, or refer to Stretches by Body Part (*see pp.156–158*). Alternatively, follow the 21-day Posture Programme (*see pp.52–65*) and compare your test results before and after.

CHEST FLEXIBILITY

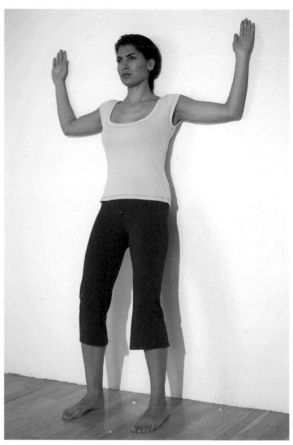

NECK FLEXIBILITY

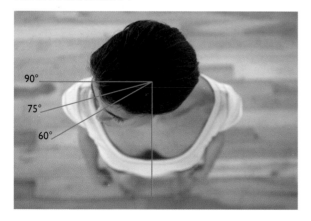

Stand with your arms by your sides, shoulders back and down, and neck relaxed. Turn your head towards your right shoulder, as far as is comfortable. Keep your gaze level; don't turn with your chin.
Less than 60° poor; 60–75° good; 75–90° very flexible

Stand with your back to a wall and take a step forwards. Position feet slightly more than hip-width apart, and lean your shoulders and head back against the wall. Bend your arms at 90° angles against the wall, elbows at shoulder height, palms facing outwards. Your forearms, upper back, and head should all touch the wall.

ARM AND SHOULDER FLEXIBILITY

Stand with back straight and shoulders back and down. Raise one arm straight up by the side of your head with palm facing inwards. Keep your hips tucked under and your abdominals tight.
Less than 160° poor; 160–180° good; 180–190° very flexible

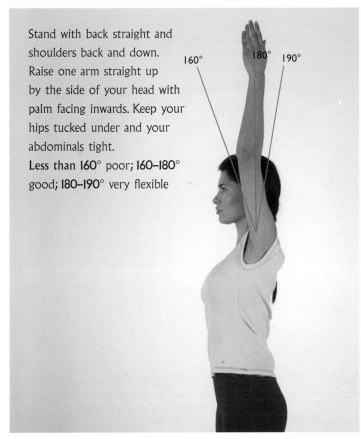

TORSO FLEXIBILITY

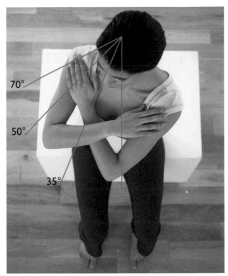

Sit forwards on a chair, back straight, and feet flat on the floor. Place your hands on opposite shoulders, and raise your elbows to chest height. Keeping your head in line with your crossed arms, turn it to the right as far as is comfortable, without moving your legs.
Less than 35° poor; 35–50° good; 50–70° very flexible

HAMSTRING FLEXIBILITY

Lie on your back, legs straight and arms at your sides. Press the calf of the bottom leg against the floor, and raise the other straight up.
Less than 75° poor; 75–90° good; 90–120° very flexible

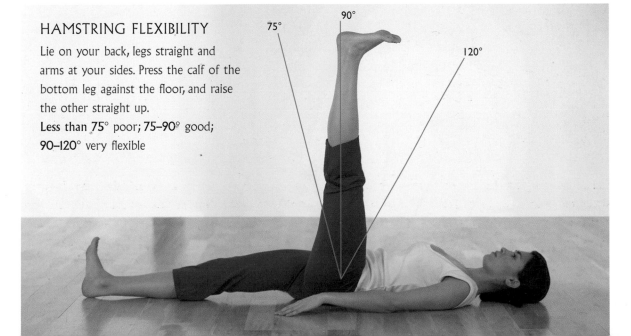

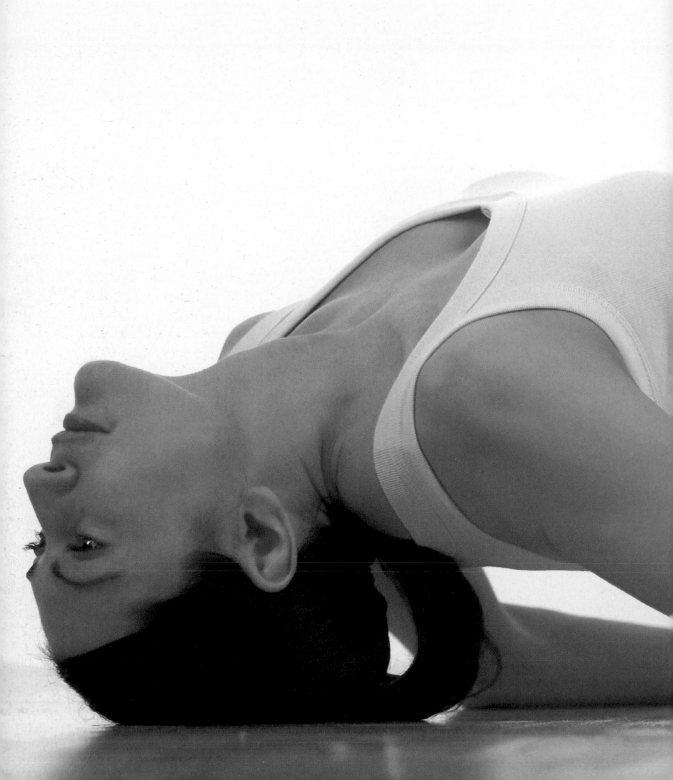

HEAD-TO-TOE CATALOGUE OF STRETCHES

There are stretches to target nearly every part of the body, from the muscles in your scalp and face that hold much of your daily tension, to the muscles and tendons in your feet that feel stiff after a long day of standing. In the pages that follow, you'll find what I consider to be key stretches, all organized by body part. Choose a stretch to suit your needs, or refer back to these stretches from the routines that appear later in the book. There are stretches for all levels of flexibility here; where possible, I've shown how to adapt positions in order to intensify a stretch.

HEAD, FACE, AND EYES

A common area of muscle stress and tension, the head and face respond favourably to attention. The scalp connects to facial and jaw muscles. The tongue, one of the most active muscles of the body, contributes to much jaw and neck discomfort, while the eyes endure constant strain. Take care when performing these stretches, and be sure to keep your head aligned over your spine.

HAIR PULL

Starting at your temples, slide your open fingers back along your scalp. Grasp a handful of hair on either side of your head and pull until you feel gentle tension on your scalp. Hold for 2 breath cycles, then release and repeat, moving around your head.

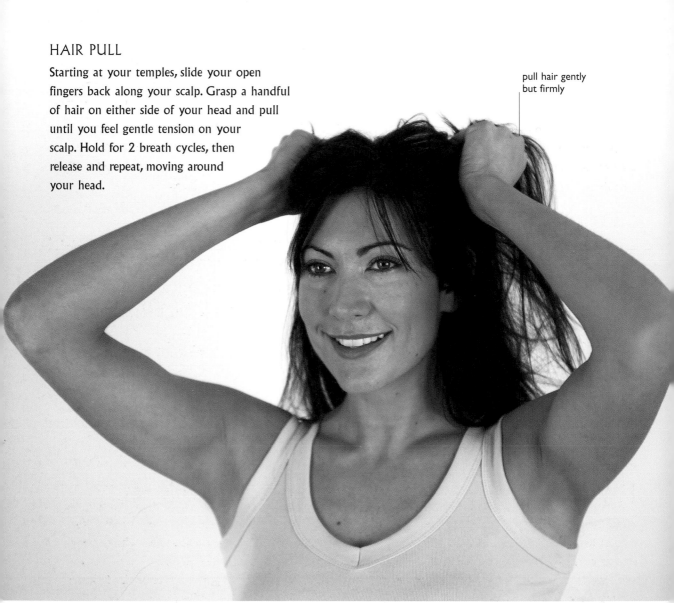

pull hair gently but firmly

LION STRETCH

This is a great stretch for the tongue, as well as the many other muscles of the face. Perform it as an end-of-day tension-reliever. Tight face and throat muscles contribute to overall tension in the rest of the body.

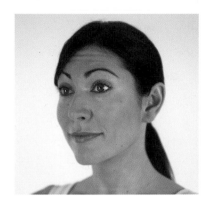

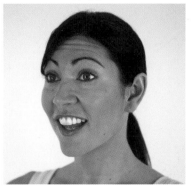

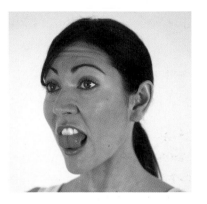

1 Raise both eyebrows as if very surprised. Lift your head, look forwards, and imagine that your ears are being pulled upwards.

2 Keep your eyebrows raised. Now open your mouth slightly and lift your top lip to expose your upper teeth.

3 Press your tongue against your lower teeth so that it pushes your jaw down. Say "ahhh" for 5 counts, then relax.

EYE STRETCHES

Be sure to keep your head still so that you isolate each of the six muscles that control the precise movements of your eyes. Perform these stretches every half hour if staring at a computer screen for long periods.

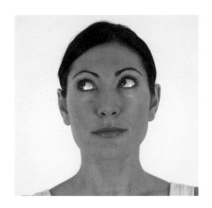

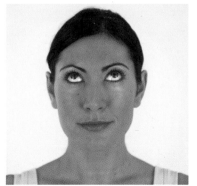

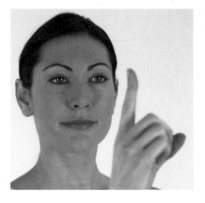

1 Focus your eyes down to the left. Follow an imaginary diagonal line up to the right, then back down to the left. Repeat 5 times. Then repeat starting at the bottom right, following the diagonal up to the left, then back down to the right.

2 Focus your eyes down to the left, then trace an imaginary horseshoe-shape up and over to the right. Then reverse the movement, starting down to the right and following the horseshoe up and over to the left. Repeat 3 more times.

3 Hold your index finger about 30 cm (1 ft) away from your nose. Stare at your fingertip for 2 breath cycles, then change your focus and look into the distance beyond your finger for 2 breath cycles. Repeat 2 more times.

NECK

The neck balances the melon-like head on the rest of the body, causing the neck muscles to work like guy-wires to support this unwieldy weight. It performs most of the twisting action of the spine and enables you to turn your head and look over your shoulder. Approach this area of the body with delicacy and precision; go slowly and take care never to pull down strongly on the head.

NECK STRETCH

After performing this sequence of neck stretches, use your hand to return your head gently to the upright position. Then soothe your neck muscles by performing what is known as a "reliever": briskly rub your hands together to generate some heat, then cup them around your neck for 5–10 seconds.

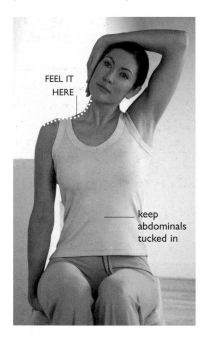

FEEL IT HERE

keep abdominals tucked in

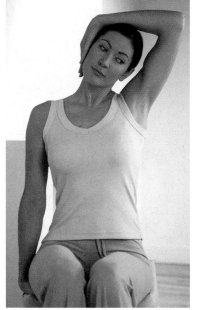

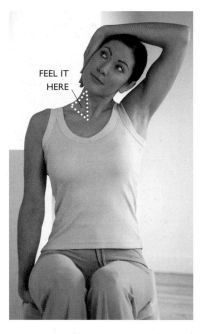

FEEL IT HERE

1 Sit slightly forwards on a chair, your feet flat on the floor. Position your right hand, palm up, under your right buttock. Drape your left arm up and over your head so that it gently tilts your head to the left. Feel a gentle stretch from your right ear to your right shoulder tip. Hold for 2 breath cycles.

2 Very slowly turn your head so that your chin faces diagonally downwards. Feel the stretch behind your right ear and down the side of your neck. Hold for 2 breath cycles, then slowly come back to centre.

3 Slowly turn your head so that your chin faces diagonally upwards. It should feel as if your eyes are being pulled upwards. Hold for 2 breath cycles, then return to the centre. Use your left hand to guide your head gently back to an upright position. Repeat steps 1–3 on the other side.

ROLL-DOWN STRETCH

The key to performing this stretch correctly is to keep your head back and your chin tucked under as you roll your head down. This ensures that you stretch the entire neck, not just the lower part of it.

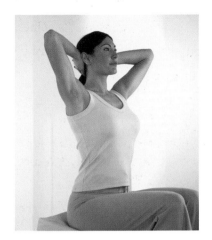

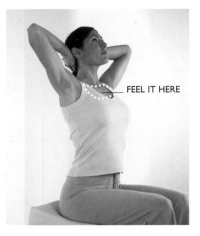

FEEL IT HERE

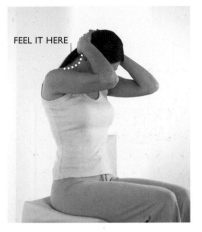

FEEL IT HERE

1 Sit slightly forwards on a chair, your feet flat on the floor. Clasp your hands behind your head and hold it as if grasping a cantaloupe with the heels of your hands. Press your head back into your hands.

2 Gently lift your gaze and look diagonally upwards. Feel as if a hook is lifting your breastbone towards the ceiling. Pull your elbows up and out as you stretch up, lifting your chest.

3 Keep the lift, and tuck your chin into your neck. Roll your head downwards to look at your chest, as if rotating your head around an axis that passes through your ears. Hold for 2 breath cycles, then roll back up.

SEATED HEAD TURN

Sit slightly forwards on a chair, your feet flat on the floor and your back straight. Turn your chin to your right shoulder. Hold on to the chair, and use your right hand to leverage more twist by pushing your right shoulder backwards. Hold for 2 breath cycles, then release and repeat on the other side.

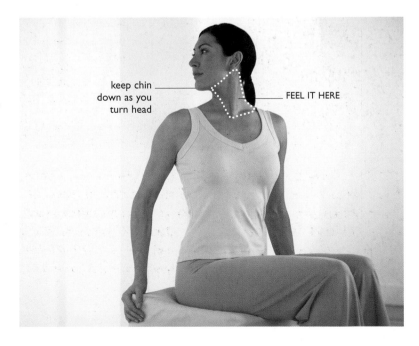

keep chin down as you turn head

FEEL IT HERE

SHOULDERS

The shoulders carry the weight of the arms and are one of the main areas of the body prone to tension. The head, neck, and shoulders all function together as a unit, so loosening up the shoulders will free up the neck, and vice versa. The stretches here will help to preserve and improve the 360° range of movement in the shoulders as well as counteract the natural tendency to hunch forwards.

SHOULDERS FRONT

This stretch helps to correct forward, slightly hunched shoulders. Perform it slowly, checking your balance and focusing the stretch by pulling your navel into your spine and holding your buttocks firm.

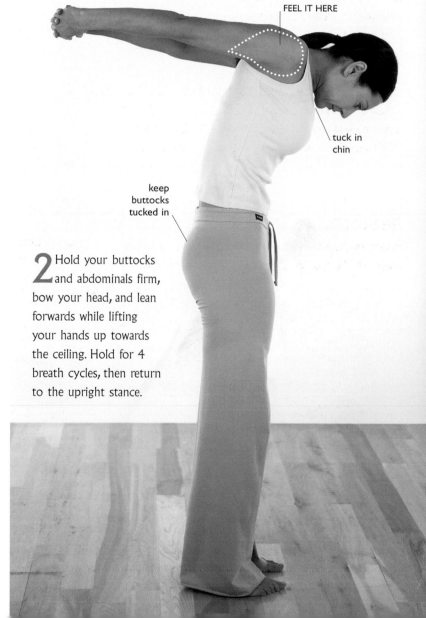

FEEL IT HERE

tuck in chin

keep buttocks tucked in

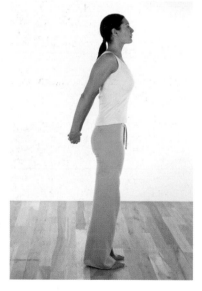

1 Stand with your hands clasped behind your back. Reach your hands away from your body and lift them slightly upwards. Be sure not to allow your upper body to tip forwards.

2 Hold your buttocks and abdominals firm, bow your head, and lean forwards while lifting your hands up towards the ceiling. Hold for 4 breath cycles, then return to the upright stance.

SHOULDERS SIDE

This stretches the muscles around the shoulder blade and in the armpit. Tightness in these areas can cause stiffness as well as restrict shoulder movements.

1 Stand with your arms extended above your head, and grasp your left wrist with your right hand. Pull the wrist upwards, elongating the left side of your body until you feel a gentle tension.

2 Maintaining the stretch, pull your left wrist up and over towards the right side. Anchor your left foot into the floor to focus the stretch. Hold for 4 breath cycles, then repeat, this time pulling your right wrist.

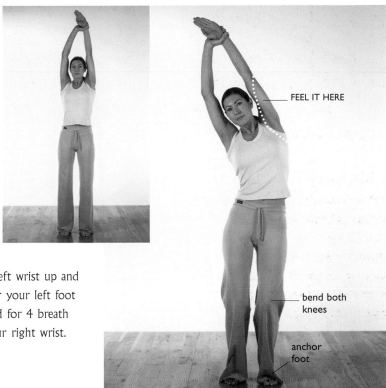

FEEL IT HERE

bend both knees

anchor foot

SHOULDERS BACK

Most people experience some muscle tightness in the backs of the shoulders. To feel the full benefit of this stretch, remember to press your neck back slightly as you tuck your chin into your chest.

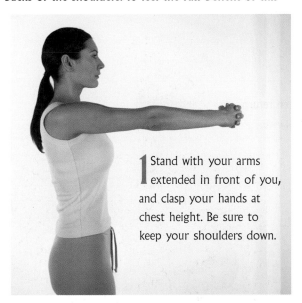

1 Stand with your arms extended in front of you, and clasp your hands at chest height. Be sure to keep your shoulders down.

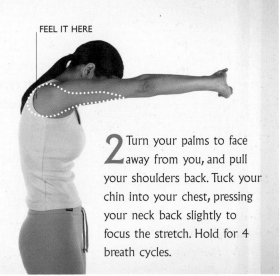

FEEL IT HERE

2 Turn your palms to face away from you, and pull your shoulders back. Tuck your chin into your chest, pressing your neck back slightly to focus the stretch. Hold for 4 breath cycles.

ARMS AND HANDS

The arms and hands perform our most mundane tasks as well as our most intricate ones. Long tendons run along the fronts and backs of the forearms to the fingers. The palms contain muscles and tendons that enable the hands to grip and the fingers to be nimble. Stretching these areas helps to relieve strain and inflammation caused by repetitive actions such as typing and knitting.

ARM STRETCH

Extend your arms in front of you at chest height and clasp your hands so that your knuckles cross. Stretch your arms by pressing the heels of your hands away from you. Focus the stretch along your arms by imagining someone pulling your shoulders back as you reach your hands forwards. Hold for 3 breath cycles.

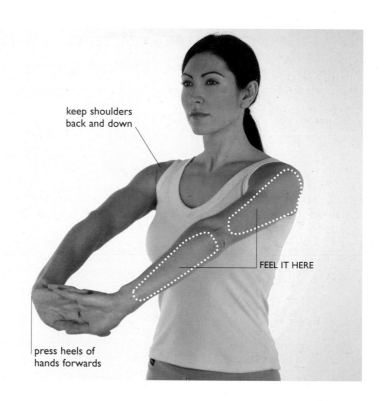

keep shoulders back and down

FEEL IT HERE

press heels of hands forwards

CLASPED FINGERS

Extend your arms in front of you at chest height. Cross your fingers at the knuckles, and turn your palms away from you. Then press your fingertips against the backs of your hands and feel the stretch in your fingers and into the palms. Hold for 3 breath cycles.

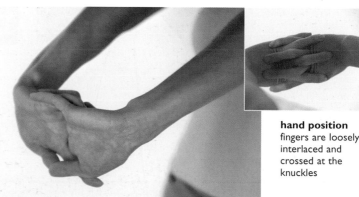

hand position fingers are loosely interlaced and crossed at the knuckles

ARMS OPEN

Stand with feet shoulder-width apart. Exhale and reach both arms upwards while pulling your shoulder blades and ribcage down. Turn your palms upwards, pressing them towards the ceiling, while reaching your fingertips down towards the floor. Feel a good stretch up through your arms but also between your ribcage and hips. Hold for 3 breath cycles.

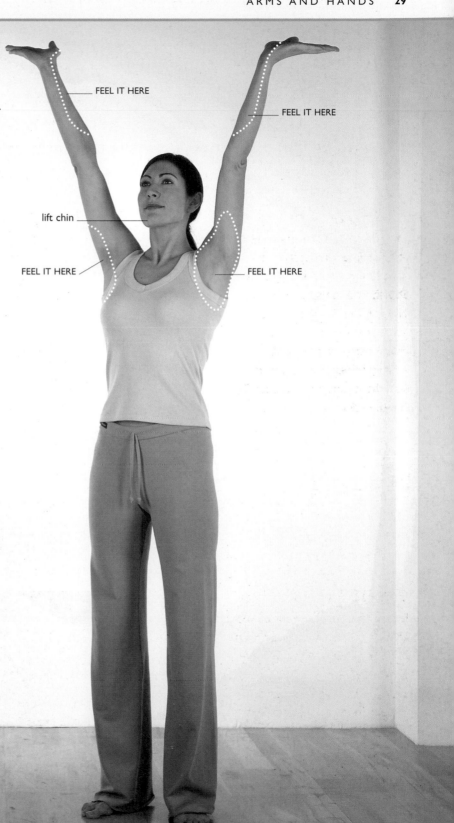

FEEL IT HERE

FEEL IT HERE

lift chin

FEEL IT HERE

FEEL IT HERE

CHEST AND RIBCAGE

We perform most of our arm movements in front of the body, which can cause the muscles of the chest to tighten as we naturally round our shoulders forwards. People who do no aerobic exercise, shallow breathers, older people, and those with asthma or breathing limitations also tend to have tight chests and ribcages. Muscle tightness in this area can also lead to arm and hand discomfort.

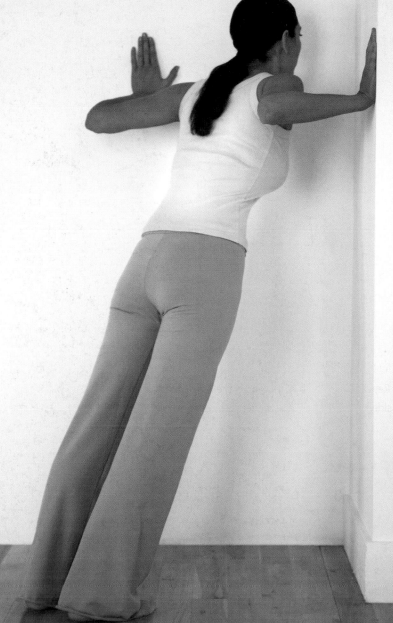

CORNER CHEST STRETCH

Stand facing a corner, hands raised at your sides, elbows bent, and hands up. Place your palms on the walls at shoulder height and lean your body weight into the corner. Pull your navel into your spine, and let your tailbone drop to focus the stretch across your chest. Hold for 4 breath cycles. This stretch can also be performed standing in a doorway.

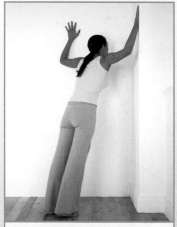

INTENSIFY THE STRETCH
Position your hands further up the walls, and reach your elbows out sideways as you lean into the corner. Feel the stretch across your shoulders and upper arms.

SINGLE ARM STRETCH

This stretches the chest muscles and the major nerves in the arms that control the precise movements of your hands. Take care; this should not be painful.

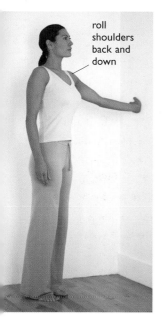

roll shoulders back and down

1 Stand facing a wall or doorway three quarters on. Place your palm on the wall midway between shoulder and waist height. Keep your elbow slightly bent to help focus the stretch on the chest and arm.

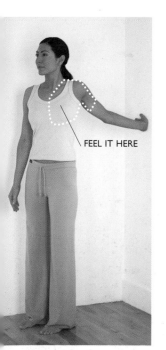

FEEL IT HERE

2 Press your hand into the wall and, feeling the stretch across your chest and in your upper arm, slowly turn away from your hand. Hold for 4 breath cycles. Repeat on the other side.

STANDING SIDE STRETCH

This stretches the sides of the ribcage while also opening up the muscles in the armpits, which have a tendency to become very tight.

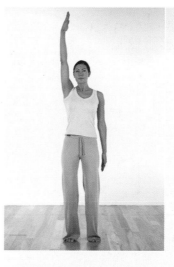

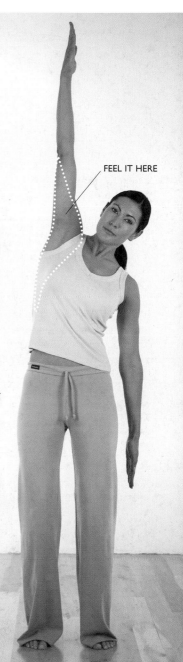

FEEL IT HERE

1 Stand with feet hip-width apart. Pull your navel into your spine, drop your tailbone, and bend your knees slightly. Raise your right arm, and stretch up as if your middle finger is being pulled towards the sky.

2 Lean to the left, pulling the left arm downwards at your side, as if your middle finger is being pulled towards the floor. Feel the stretch in the right side of your ribcage. Hold for 4 breath cycles., then repeat on the other side.

UPPER BACK

The muscles in the upper back are in constant use as they help to stabilize the body when we move our arms; they must also manoeuvre the weight of the head. Ideally, aim to stretch this area of the body several times a day as this helps to loosen up the head, neck, and arms to work together in smooth co-ordination. Pay attention to form in order to isolate the upper back and protect the spine.

UPPER BACK FORWARD STRETCH

The key to this stretch is to tuck your chin in and imagine that an axis runs through your ears as you tilt your head forwards. This is a delicate part of the body, so perform this stretch slowly, rolling down your spine as you lower your head. This stretch can bring enormous relief after long periods sitting or driving.

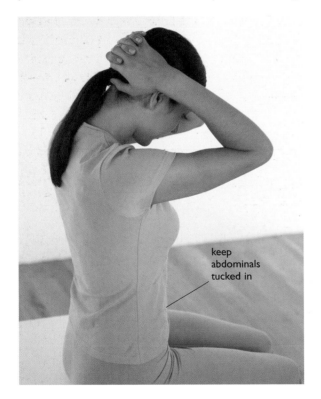

keep abdominals tucked in

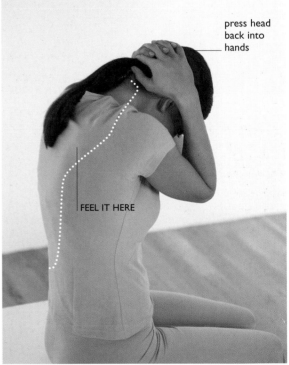

press head back into hands

FEEL IT HERE

1 Sit slightly forwards on the edge of a chair and clasp your hands behind your head. Fold your arms so that your elbows point forwards, and tuck your chin into your chest. Keeping your abdominals tucked in, slowly rotate your head downwards, imagining that an axis runs through your ears.

2 Keep your chin tucked into your chest as you roll your head downwards while gently pressing your head back into your hands. Cave your chest and look at your breastbone. Feel a good stretch from your neck down through your upper back and hold for 2 breath cycles. Then slowly roll your head back up.

TWIST, ARMS CROSSED

Be sure to keep your head back and aligned over your pelvis so that you are sitting up tall as you perform this stretch. Keep your shoulders down as you twist. Imagine that your spine is a long towel twisting upon itself. Feel the long strips of muscle along the sides of the spine working.

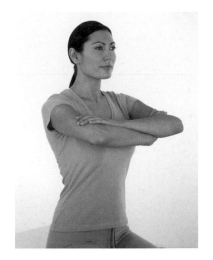 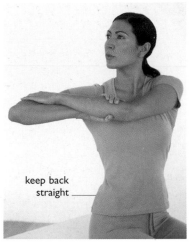

keep back straight

1 Sit slightly forwards on a chair, your feet flat on the floor. Cross your arms in front of you, and lift your elbows slightly so that they are just below chest height.

2 Exhale as you twist to the right and use your right hand to pull your left forearm around yourself. Look to the right. Hold for 2 breath cycles, then return to the forward position. Repeat on the other side.

SEATED TWIST

In this exercise, you push with one arm to leverage the twist and really stretch the spine. Protect your spine by pulling your abdomen in deeply as you try to maintain the longest vertical height. Only go as far as is comfortable. Feel a good stretch between and just below your shoulder blades.

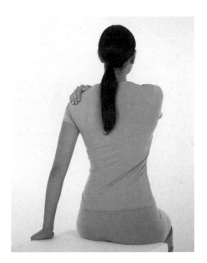 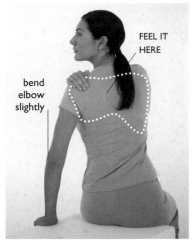

FEEL IT HERE

bend elbow slightly

1 Sit slightly forwards on a chair, your feet flat on the floor. Cross your right hand over and hold on to your left shoulder. Hold the edge of the seat (or arm of a chair) with your left hand.

2 Twist to the left, increasing the stretch by pushing forwards with your left hand on the seat. Pull your left shoulder back and hold for 2 breath cycles, then relax out of the stretch and repeat on the other side.

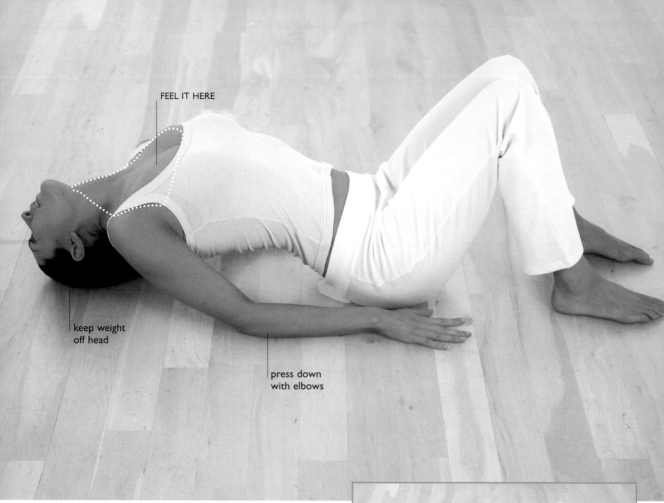

FEEL IT HERE

keep weight
off head

press down
with elbows

THE FISH

Lie on your back with knees bent, soles of your feet
on the floor, and arms by your sides with palms facing
down. Pull your navel into your spine and arch your
lower back upwards. Press down on your elbows and
slide your head in, arching your upper body. Feel the
muscles between your shoulder blades working, as well
as the stretch across your upper chest. Hold for 2
breath cycles, then support yourself on your elbows as
you slide your head out and straighten your back on
the floor.

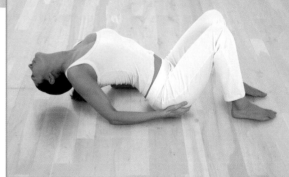

INTENSIFY THE STRETCH

Grab your buttocks, arch your back up, roll your shoulders
back, and tuck your elbows in. Gently lift your head off the
floor and feel an increased stretch in your upper back, across
your chest, and in the front of your neck. Slowly release by
lowering your head to the floor and straightening your back.

HIPS UP

This stretch is great for opening a tight upper back. The key is to keep your chin tucked into your chest as you roll your head forwards. You might want to place a cushion or folded towel under your knees to make this position more comfortable. Be sure to roll forwards slowly to keep balance and form.

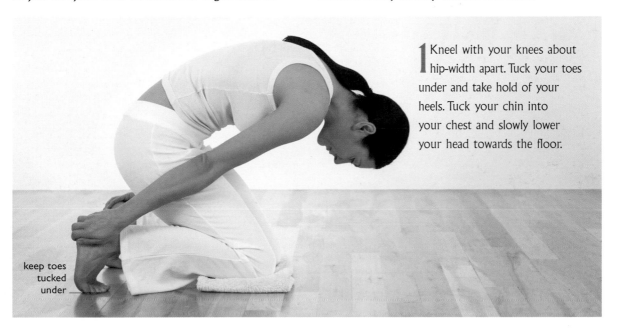

1 Kneel with your knees about hip-width apart. Tuck your toes under and take hold of your heels. Tuck your chin into your chest and slowly lower your head towards the floor.

keep toes tucked under

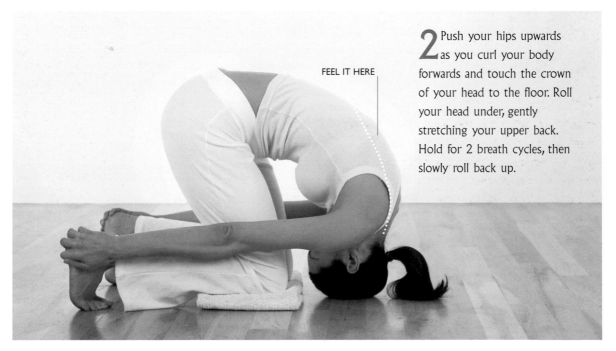

FEEL IT HERE

2 Push your hips upwards as you curl your body forwards and touch the crown of your head to the floor. Roll your head under, gently stretching your upper back. Hold for 2 breath cycles, then slowly roll back up.

LOWER BACK

A strong lower back keeps us upright against the force of gravity and also functions as a shock absorber, softening the impact when our feet hit the ground. Both prolonged sitting and standing can tighten and stiffen the lower back muscles. These stretches will improve suppleness and relieve muscle stiffness. If you experience discomfort when performing a stretch, come out of it immediately.

SEATED HEAD CURL

This is a good basic back stretch that you can do anywhere there's a chair. Curve your back by pulling your navel into your spine as you roll your head towards your knees. Think of your pelvis anchoring down into the seat and the crown of your head reaching up and over a fence to help you to round your back.

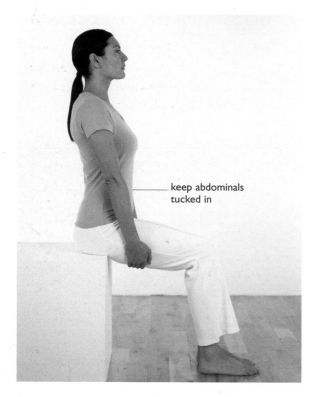

keep abdominals tucked in

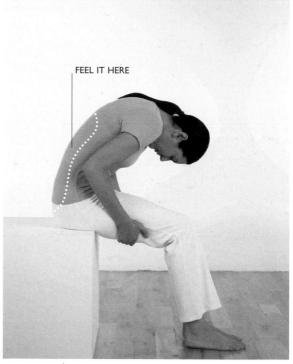

FEEL IT HERE

1 Sit slightly forwards on a chair, your feet flat on the floor. Sit up straight, tighten your abdominals, and grasp the backs of your thighs.

2 Tuck your chin into your chest, rotating your head down as if an imaginary axis runs through your ears. Round your back, caving your chest, and gently pull with your arms to curl your head towards your knees. Pull your navel into your spine and hold for 2 breath cycles. Slowly uncurl to the upright sitting position.

KNEES TO CHEST

Another basic back stretch, the key again is to tuck your chin into your chest as you curl up and pull your abdominals in. Imagine making yourself into a perfectly round ball. You might want to place a folded towel or pillow under your shoulders to make this stretch more comfortable.

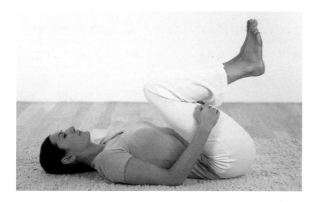

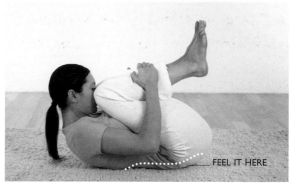

FEEL IT HERE

1 Lie on your back with your knees bent. Tighten your abdominals and lift your thighs towards your chest. Gently press your lower back into the floor as you reach forwards and grasp your thighs.

2 Exhale and gently tuck your chin into your chest as you take hold of your shins and curl your head forwards. Bring your shoulders towards your heels, and hold for 2 breath cycles, then relax down.

FEET OVER HEAD

Lie on your back. Bend your knees and, controlling the movement with your abdominals, slowly bring your feet up and back over your head so that they touch the floor behind you. Gently pull your calves with your hands. Find a comfortable position and hold for 2 breath cycles. Then slowly roll down, bringing your feet back to the floor.

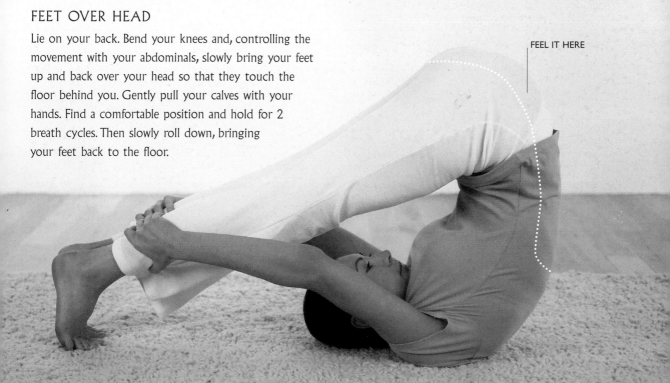

FEEL IT HERE

FEEL IT HERE

round back

keep
abdominals
tucked in

bend knees
slightly

HANGING WITH CROSSED ARMS

Pull your navel into your spine, lift your pelvic floor, and exhale as you tuck your chin into your chest and roll down to a comfortable position. Cross your arms and hold on to your upper arms or elbows. Round your back so that you are looking at your navel. Don't allow yourself to tip forwards. Hold for 2 breath cycles, then slowly roll back up.

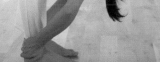

FEEL IT HERE

INTENSIFY THE STRETCH
Tighten your abdominals to pull your head in closer to your legs, and hold on to your ankles. Feel a good stretch down through your buttocks.

CROSSOVER REACH BACK

This advanced stretch opens both the lower back and the deep muscles of the pelvis. Be sure to hold your abdominals firmly into the spine and to keep the groin lifted for support throughout the whole stretch. Come out of the stretch immediately if you experience any dizziness or if you feel light-headed.

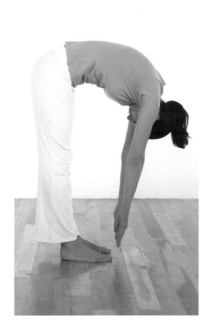

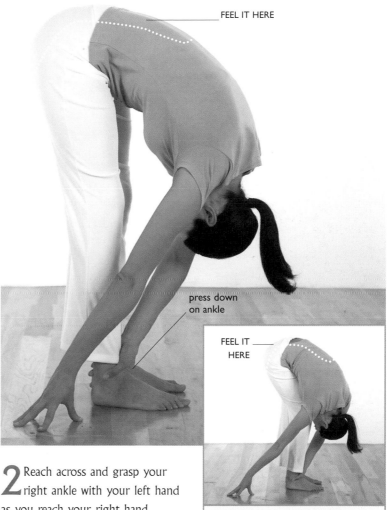

FEEL IT HERE

press down on ankle

FEEL IT HERE

1 Stand with your feet about hip-width apart. Exhale as you tuck your chin into your chest, bend your knees slightly, and roll your spine down to a comfortable position. Reach down with your arms. Be sure to keep your abdominals tucked in.

2 Reach across and grasp your right ankle with your left hand as you reach your right hand behind you towards the floor. Press down with your left hand to help support your hanging body weight. Hold for 2 breath cycles, then use your hands to help you to roll back up to upright. Repeat the stretch on the other side.

INTENSIFY THE STRETCH
Reach back with your right arm, touching the floor with your fingertips. Exhale and bend your right knee slightly. Inhale, then exhale and walk your right fingertips further behind you. Inhale, then exhale and walk your fingertips a little further. Feel the stretch in your buttocks. Finally, exhale, release your arm hold, and roll up.

WAIST

The corset-like muscles of the waist protect the vital organs, support the spine, and connect the upper and lower bodies. The waist is the malleable part of the torso that enables the bony structures of the ribcage and pelvis to twist in different directions. The waist has a tendency to slump and collapse; regular stretching can help to lengthen the muscles so that they can be properly strengthened.

STANDING WAIST TWIST

Stand with feet about hip-width apart. Place your right hand, fingers pointing down, firmly on the right side of your lower back. Pull your navel into your spine and, leading with your left hand, twist diagonally up and around to the right. Feel a good stretch in the left side of your waist and up the body. Hold for 2 breath cycles, then release. Repeat, twisting to the other side.

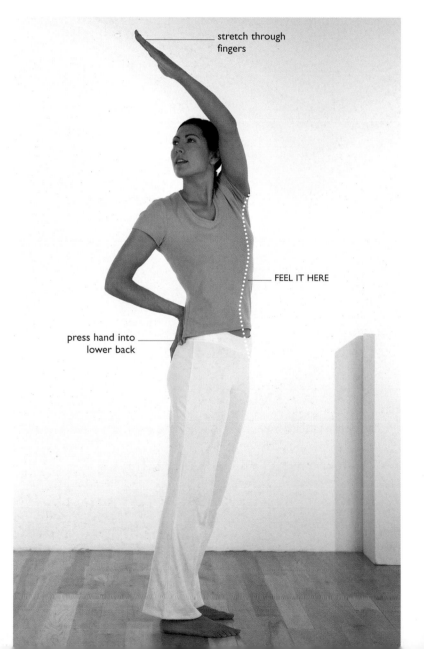

stretch through fingers

FEEL IT HERE

press hand into lower back

SEATED WAIST STRETCH

To get the full benefit of this stretch, elongate both sides of the torso as you reach up. Focus on stretching up and then over as you reach to the side. Gaze ahead and hold yourself back to keep from leaning forwards.

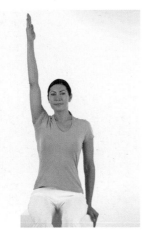

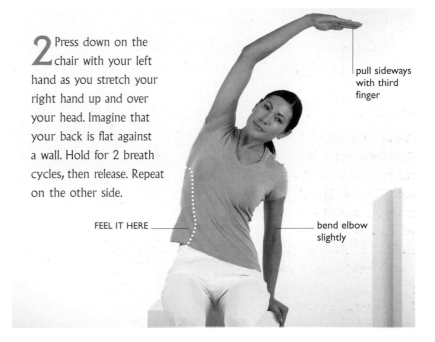

2 Press down on the chair with your left hand as you stretch your right hand up and over your head. Imagine that your back is flat against a wall. Hold for 2 breath cycles, then release. Repeat on the other side.

pull sideways with third finger

FEEL IT HERE

bend elbow slightly

1 Sit slightly forwards on a chair, feet flat on the floor. Reach up with your right hand; hold on to the chair with your left hand.

LYING WAIST TWIST

Lie on your back. Extend your arms at your sides, and hold your abdominals firm as you cross your right knee over towards the floor on your left side. Bend your left leg slightly. Press your right knee towards the floor while pushing your right hip forwards. Hold for 2 breath cycles, then gently release and repeat on the other side.

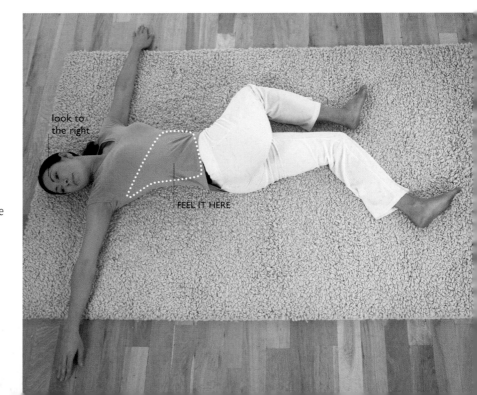

look to the right

FEEL IT HERE

HIPS

The muscles surrounding the hip joints and pelvis are dense due to the fact that they must bear the weight of the entire upper body. We have both deep hip flexors, muscles that run from the front of the spine to the top inner thigh, and superficial hip flexors, which run from the hip bone to the knee. Walking develops these muscles, and they benefit greatly from being stretched.

FRONT HIP STRETCH

This stretch targets both the deep and the superficial hip flexors. Feel it by tucking your pelvis under.

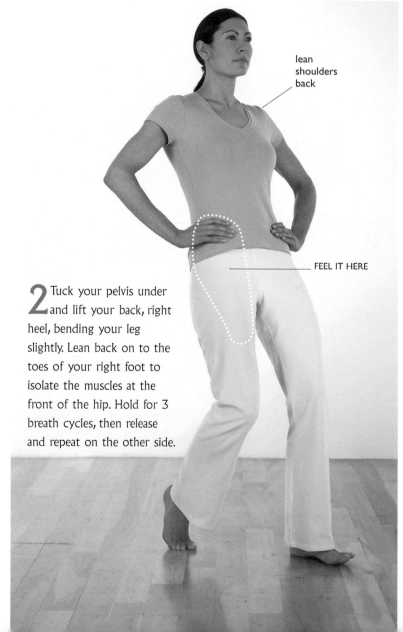

lean shoulders back

FEEL IT HERE

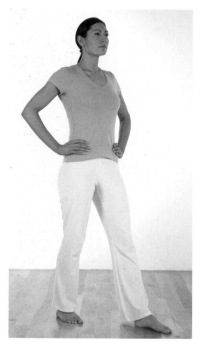

1 Place you hands on your hips, and step forwards with your left foot. Stand with one leg forward, both knees slightly bent.

2 Tuck your pelvis under and lift your back, right heel, bending your leg slightly. Lean back on to the toes of your right foot to isolate the muscles at the front of the hip. Hold for 3 breath cycles, then release and repeat on the other side.

SIDE HIP STRETCH

Stand with your left leg crossed in front of your right, the toes of your left foot touching the floor. Raise your right arm up, and place your left hand on the left side of your pelvis. Tighten your abdominals and stretch over to the left as you push in with your left hand. Feel the stretch in the right side of your pelvis. Hold for 4 breath cycles, then release and repeat on the other side.

LEG-CROSS HIP STRETCH

This stretch targets the muscles around the hip joints. It helps to improve flexibility and strength necessary for hip stability.

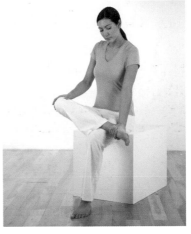

1 Sit comfortably with your legs crossed so that your right ankle is on your left thigh.

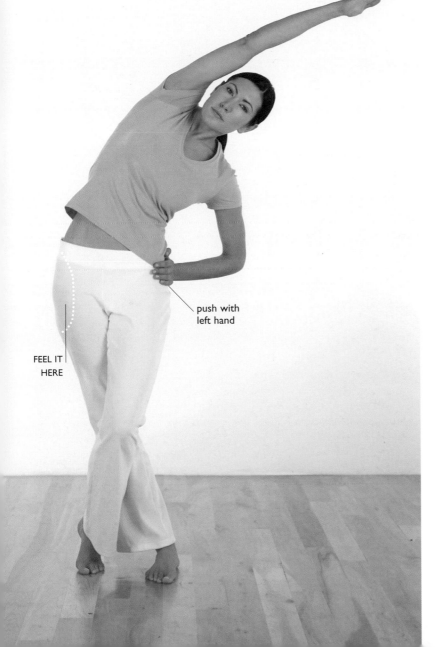

push with left hand

FEEL IT HERE

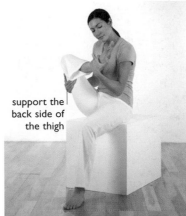

support the back side of the thigh

2 Pull your right ankle towards your left shoulder. Feel the stretch on the outside of your right hip and hold for 4 breath cycles. Release, and repeat on the other side.

THIGHS

The large muscles on the tops of the thighs, the quadriceps (quads), are called the bully of the body because they tend to dominate leg movements. Tight quads can cause painful knees, while the hamstrings in the backs of the thighs tend to cause lower back problems if they are not stretched. The inner thighs help to support the spine; it is essential that they are stretched and equally balanced too.

STANDING QUAD STRETCH

This is the basic quad stretch. Keep your bent knee aligned under your pelvis, and be careful not to let it veer to the side. As you stretch, avoid pulling too hard on the foot – you should not experience any knee pain. If you have difficulty balancing, rest your free hand on a wall or chair for support.

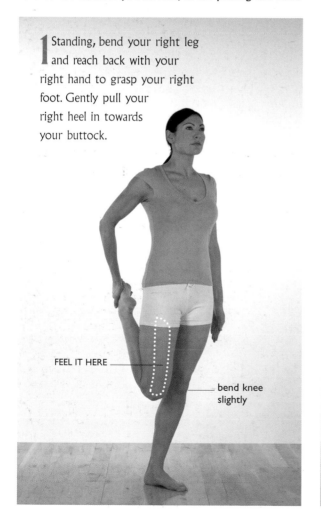

1 Standing, bend your right leg and reach back with your right hand to grasp your right foot. Gently pull your right heel in towards your buttock.

FEEL IT HERE

bend knee slightly

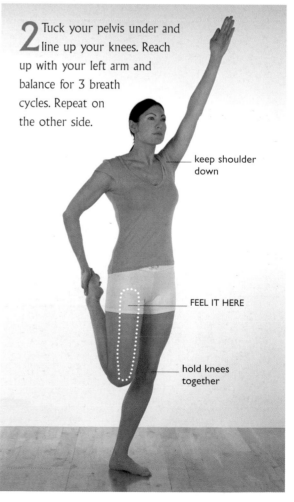

2 Tuck your pelvis under and line up your knees. Reach up with your left arm and balance for 3 breath cycles. Repeat on the other side.

keep shoulder down

FEEL IT HERE

hold knees together

INNER THIGH SQUAT

Stand with feet a little wider than shoulder-width apart, toes pointing slightly outwards. Place your hands on your thighs for support, and squat down, tucking your pelvis under. Feel a good stretch across both inner thighs and hold for 3 breath cycles.

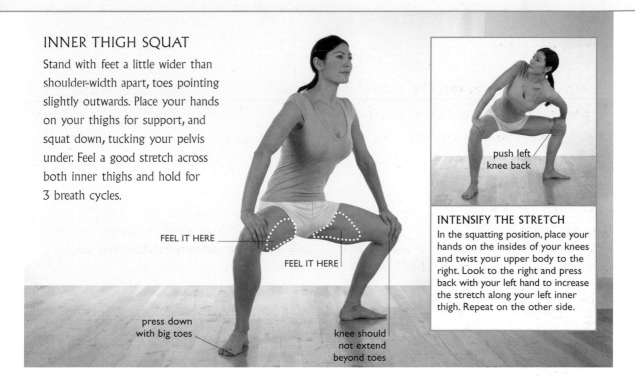

push left knee back

FEEL IT HERE

FEEL IT HERE

press down with big toes

knee should not extend beyond toes

INTENSIFY THE STRETCH

In the squatting position, place your hands on the insides of your knees and twist your upper body to the right. Look to the right and press back with your left hand to increase the stretch along your left inner thigh. Repeat on the other side.

OUTER THIGH STRETCH

This slightly more advanced stretch is sometimes easier to perform sitting on a large book such as a telephone directory or a short stool. It stretches the abductors, the muscles on the outsides of the thighs.

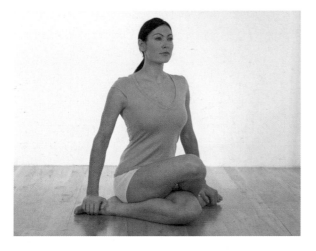

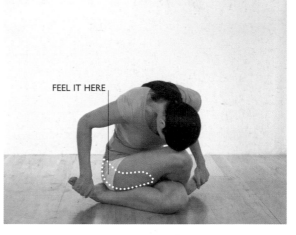

FEEL IT HERE

1 Sit comfortably with your legs crossed. If you can, line your knees up on top of each other. Firmly grasp a foot in each hand. Take care to cross your legs only as far as is comfortable.

2 Gently pull up and back on your feet, and bend your head slightly forwards, if you can. Feel a strong stretch along the side of your top leg. Hold for 4 breath cycles. Repeat with your legs crossed the other way.

STANDING HAMSTRING STRETCH

Stand on your left foot and place the heel of your right foot ahead of you. Tilt your torso forwards and place your hands just above your right knee. Pull your navel into your spine and flatten your back until you feel the stretch in the back of your right thigh. Hold for 3 breath cycles, then release and repeat on the other side.

SUPPORTED HAMSTRING STRETCH

Stand on your left foot and place your right heel on a support that is ideally no higher than mid-thigh. The knee of your raised leg should be comfortable for this advanced stretch. Place your hands on your right thigh, lengthen your torso, and lean forwards over your propped up leg. Hold for 4 breath cycles. Release and repeat on the other side.

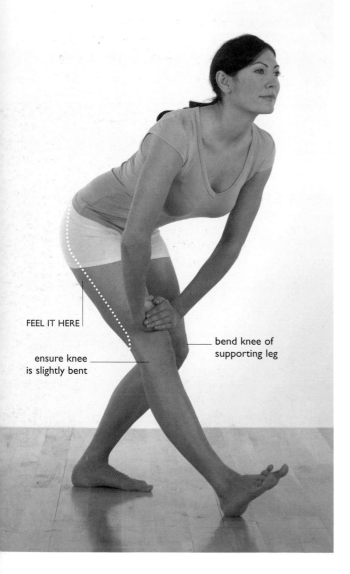

FEEL IT HERE

ensure knee is slightly bent

bend knee of supporting leg

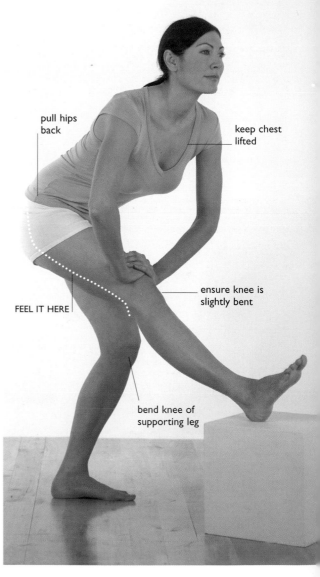

pull hips back

keep chest lifted

ensure knee is slightly bent

FEEL IT HERE

bend knee of supporting leg

LYING HAMSTRING STRETCH

Step 1 provides a simple and effective hamstring stretch and can be performed on its own, if preferred. Step 2 intensifies the stretch slightly. Remember to pull your abdominals in to support your back.

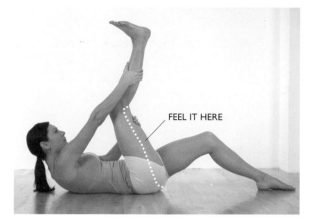

FEEL IT HERE

1 Lie down and gently pull your right leg towards you with your left leg slightly bent on the floor. Tuck your chin into your chest to help support your neck and spine, and flatten your abdominals, pulling them in. If performing just this step of the stretch, hold for 4 breath cycles, then release and repeat on the other leg.

2 Straighten your left leg on the floor, and press your calf down as you gently pull your right thigh towards you. Lower your head to the floor. Hold for 4 breath cycles, then release and repeat on the other leg.

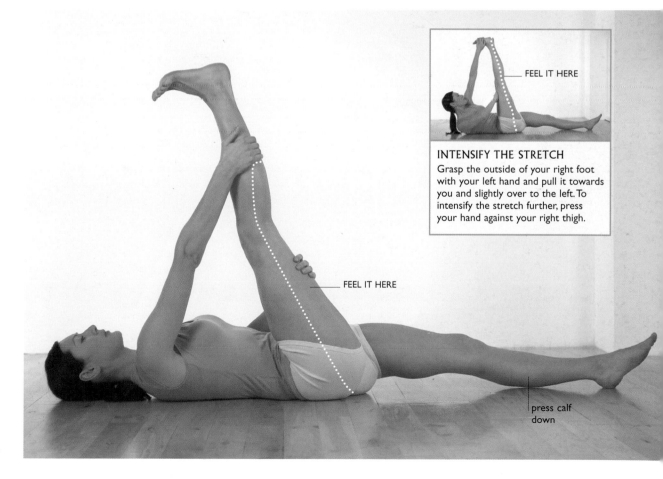

FEEL IT HERE

INTENSIFY THE STRETCH
Grasp the outside of your right foot with your left hand and pull it towards you and slightly over to the left. To intensify the stretch further, press your hand against your right thigh.

FEEL IT HERE

press calf down

CALVES

The calves become tight from the strain of working to hold us up when we are standing and then shortening as we sit or lie down. Tight calves may contribute to lower back problems as well as Achilles' tendon and foot complaints. You need to perform two exercises to stretch the calf muscle fully as it consists of two parts, one originating from above the knee, the other from below it.

BASIC LUNGE

The key to this stretch is to ensure that your tailbone points down towards the floor and not to the back heel as you lunge.

2 Bend your left leg but don't allow the knee to extend beyond your toes. Gently shift your weight forwards, keeping your right heel on the floor. Hold the stretch for 4 breath cycles, then release. Repeat with your right leg stepped forwards.

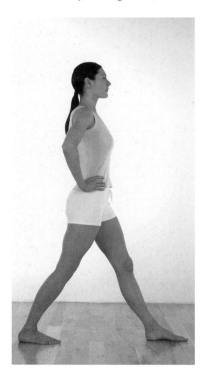

1 Place your hands on your hips, and take a large step forwards with your left foot. Be sure to keep your back straight and your shoulders back and down.

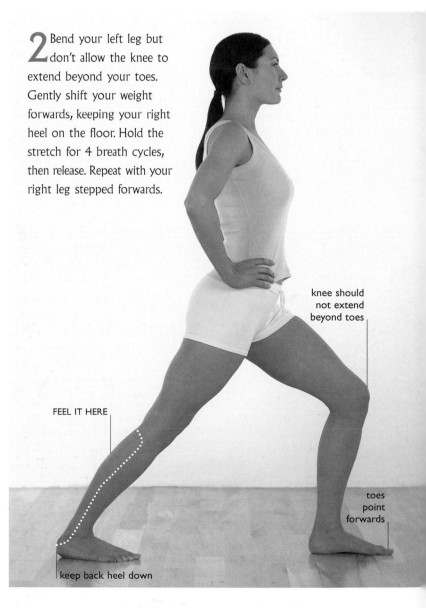

knee should not extend beyond toes

FEEL IT HERE

toes point forwards

keep back heel down

STEP DROP

This targets the soleus, the bottom calf muscle that runs into the Achilles' tendon, and can help to prevent injury there.

2 Slowly lower your heels below the step line until you feel a good stretch in your lower calves. Hold for 4 breath cycles.

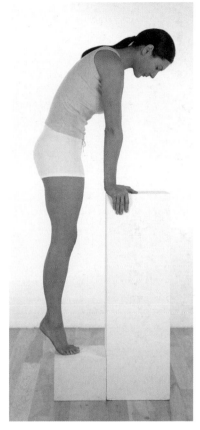

1 Stand with your toes and the balls of your feet on a step, your weight forwards. Hold on to a support for balance, if needed. Lift your heels as high as you can.

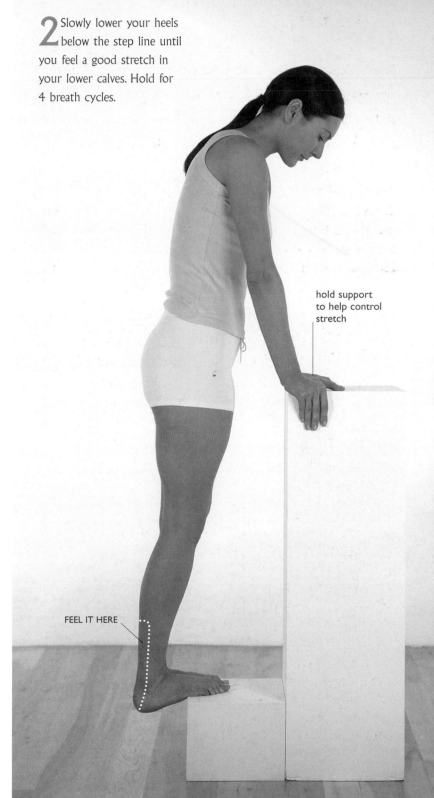

hold support to help control stretch

FEEL IT HERE

ANKLES AND FEET

An often neglected area of the body, our overused ankles and feet benefit from regular stretching. The foot is made up of 26 bones, and the sole has four layers of muscles and tendons. As we know from reflexology, stretching the soles of the feet can affect the whole body, from the internal organs to the musculoskeletal system. Stretching the feet can help to relieve muscle tension in the hips.

FOOT POINTER

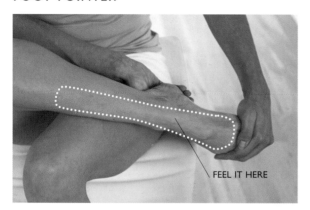

FEEL IT HERE

Sit comfortably with one leg crossed over the other so that you can reach your foot. Grasp the front of your foot with one hand. Elongate the top of the foot away from the shinbone while gently pressing the heel up into the back of the calf. Feel the front of the ankle opening up, and hold for 4 breath cycles. Release and repeat on the other foot.

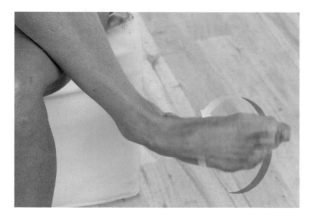

SIDE FOOT STRETCH

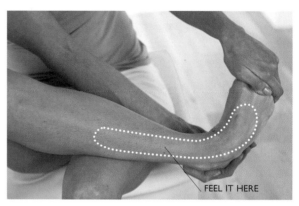

FEEL IT HERE

Sit comfortably with one leg crossed over the other. Gently grasp the front of your foot and pull your toes in towards you. Hold for 3 breath cycles, then press your toes away from you, again holding the stretch for 3 breath cycles. Release and repeat on the other foot.

ANKLE CIRCLES

Sit or stand to perform this stretch. Moving clockwise, slowly trace the shape of a large circle with your toes. Circle your foot 5 times clockwise, then repeat, circling anticlockwise. Perform large circular motions. Repeat with the other foot.

TRANSVERSE ARCH

You should be able to bend your toes to expose your knuckles, just as you do on your hand when you make a fist. The knuckles on your toes should slope down, with the big toe knuckle the highest and the little toe the lowest. Here you position your fingers under the foot and stretch the top and then the bottom of it.

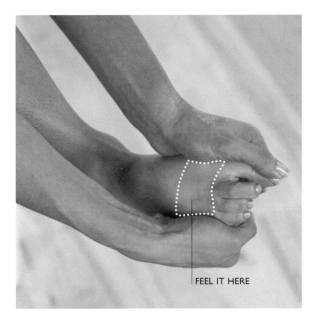

FEEL IT HERE

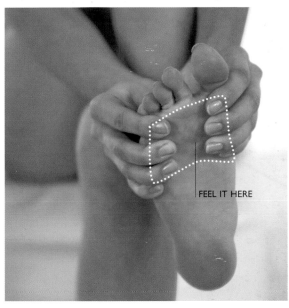

FEEL IT HERE

1 Grasp your foot with both hands so that your fingers meet under your knuckle arch. Slowly and firmly spread the knuckles apart as you apply upwards pressure with your fingers. Repeat 5 times.

2 Position your thumbs next to each other on top of your foot. Press down firmly as you open and stretch the bottom of your foot with your fingers. Do this 5 times. Repeat both steps on the other foot.

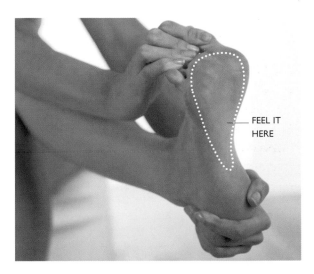

FEEL IT HERE

TOE BEND

Sit comfortably and lift your foot so that the sole faces away from you. Grasp your heel to keep your foot steady, and firmly pull your toes up towards your shin. Tuck your fingers under the pads of your toes and pull and lengthen rather than just bending your toes back. Hold for 3 breath cycles, then repeat on the other foot.

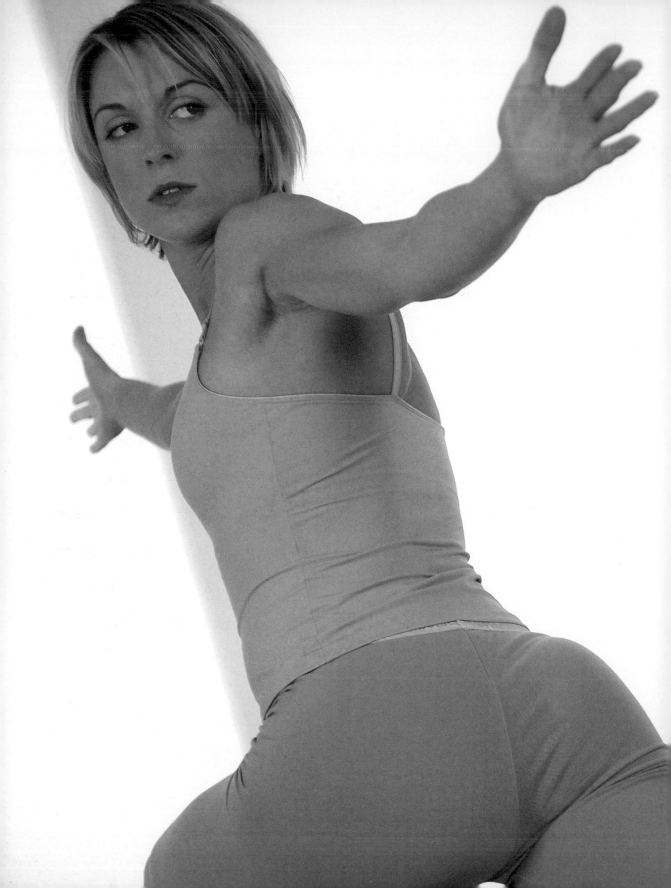

21-DAY POSTURE PROGRAMME

We carry heavy bags, hunch over desks, work at computers, and hold our bodies in awkward positions. Most of our day-to-day activities are performed with our arms and hands — in front of us — which accentuates our natural tendency to hunch forwards. Posture deteriorates as the framework of our muscles is slowly pulled out of alignment. But help is at hand. Follow this simple programme and learn how a short, daily stretching routine can rebalance your muscles and help to achieve a straighter, sleeker, and more dynamic you.

USING THE PROGRAMME

The programme's ultimate goal is to produce the tallest, most vertical you that is possible. It targets typical problem areas by rebalancing and reconditioning your muscles, helping you to achieve your ideal posture (*see pp.10–11*). Set aside just 15 minutes every day and you'll be amazed by what you can achieve – by how different you not only feel but look by the end of the programme. You will notice the effects immediately, but they will last and only improve over time.

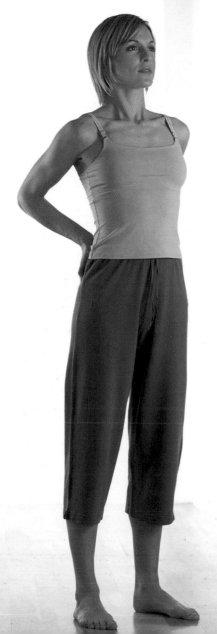

Studies have shown that bad postural habits can be relearned. By following the programme, you can achieve a visible improvement in posture in just three weeks. The programme focuses on typical postural problems, most of which can be corrected with simple stretches that balance the muscles. Stretches that open the chest, tighten the abdominals, and lengthen the lower back counteract the body's natural tendency to hunch the shoulders forwards and slouch. You will learn how to sit and stand with correct posture, as well as improve general muscle flexibility.

Getting results

The key to success is to take the programme into your daily life as well as setting aside time to do your routine every day. Perform each routine at least once daily – it should only take about 15 minutes. Then reinforce the programme by using the week's cue to prompt you to check your posture as you go about your daily activities. The cueing technique teaches you body awareness, so you train your mind to strive for good posture as well as your body.

If possible, ask someone to take a picture of you in profile on day one of the programme. Then ask them to take a final picture on day 21 and compare the two. You can't fail to be impressed by the improvement.

Muscle balancing can bring about dramatic improvements in posture. Check your posture constantly, and correct the inevitable tendency to slump forwards. Stand straight; sit tall.

WEEK ONE

These seated stretches address the body's tendency to hunch forwards and will help to encourage good posture when sitting. Keep your head aligned over your pelvis and your shoulders back and down. Begin by sitting slightly forwards on a chair, your feet flat on the floor. Allow 15 minutes to complete this routine.

WEEK ONE CUE

Imagine that your head is a bowling ball. This week, every time that you eat, practise balancing this bowling ball on top of a long giraffe neck. Be aware of the slight nuances that a head tilt can create, and how other body parts feel as a result.

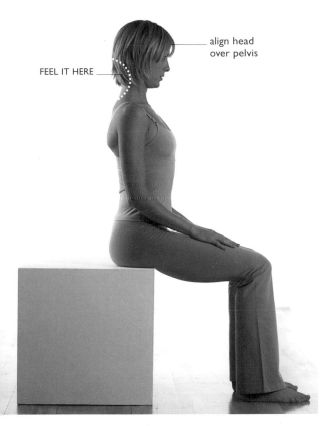

align head over pelvis

FEEL IT HERE

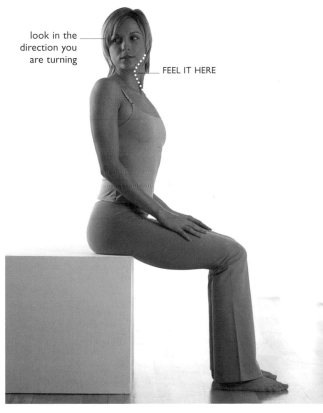

look in the direction you are turning

FEEL IT HERE

1 Sit up straight and place your hands on your thighs. Open your chest by pulling your shoulders back and down. Keep your head aligned over your pelvis and bring your ears back, dropping your chin slightly. Gently press the back of your neck against an imaginary wall while at the same time sliding your head upwards. Hold for 4 breath cycles, then relax.

2 With your head aligned over your pelvis and your chin on the same level, turn your head towards your right shoulder. Feel every degree of the rotation, and make the turn as smooth and circular as possible. Go as far as is comfortable. Look to the right. Hold for 4 breath cycles, then repeat, turning your head to the left. Return to centre.

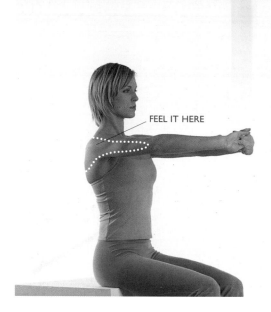

FEEL IT HERE

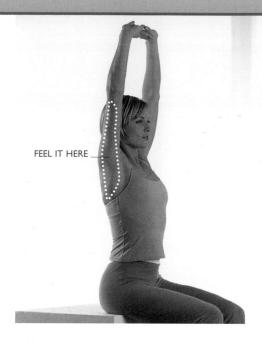

FEEL IT HERE

3 Clasp your hands in front of you: if you normally place your right index finger over your left, reverse it here. Push forwards, palms facing out. Hold for 4 breath cycles; stretch a little further forwards with each breath.

4 Inhale and reach your arms overhead. Try to keep your shoulders down and away from your ears. Press your palms up towards the ceiling for 4 breath cycles; try to stretch a little further up with each breath.

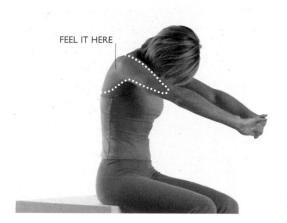

FEEL IT HERE

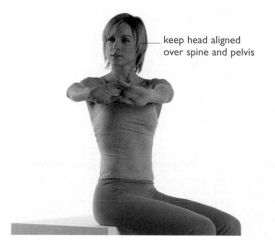

keep head aligned over spine and pelvis

5 Lower your hands so that they are just below chest level, palms still turned outwards. Gently tilt your chin down, imagining an axis that runs from ear to ear, and look towards your navel. Press your hands outwards and slightly down, feeling the stretch in your shoulders and across your upper back. Hold for 4 breath cycles.

6 With fingers still clasped and palms out-turned, raise your hands to chest level in front of you. Keeping your head aligned over your pelvis, twist around to the right. Move your hands to the right, letting your right fingers squeeze and pull your left hand to the right. Hold for 4 breath cycles, then repeat on the left side.

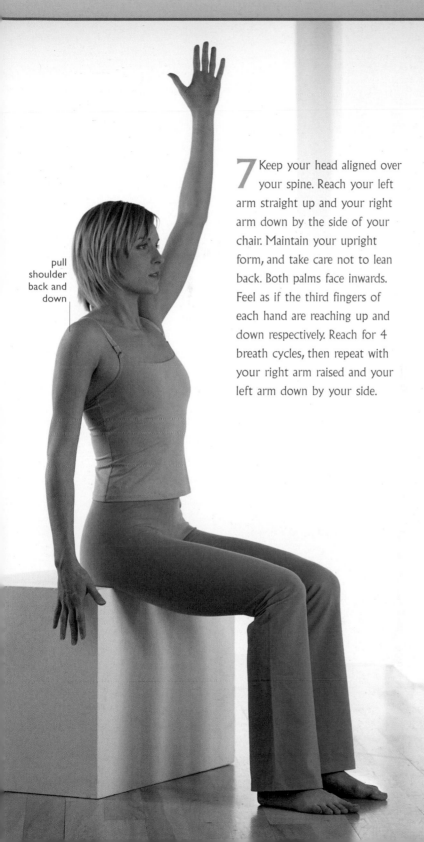

pull shoulder back and down

7 Keep your head aligned over your spine. Reach your left arm straight up and your right arm down by the side of your chair. Maintain your upright form, and take care not to lean back. Both palms face inwards. Feel as if the third fingers of each hand are reaching up and down respectively. Reach for 4 breath cycles, then repeat with your right arm raised and your left arm down by your side.

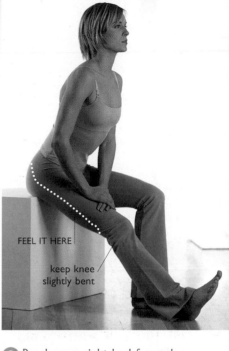

FEEL IT HERE

keep knee slightly bent

8 Reach your right heel forwards on the floor in front of you and point your toes up. Place your hands on your thigh. Keep your back flat, and lean forwards slightly over your outstretched leg, tilting from your hips. Feel the stretch behind the buttocks and in the back of your outstretched leg. Hold for 4 breath cycles, then repeat on the other side.

WEEK TWO

In Week One, you learned awareness of your body when sitting. Now we bring that awareness to standing. In Week Two, continue with the seated exercises from Week One, but add this five-minute sequence of standing stretches. These exercises encourage proper alignment of the head, spine, and pelvis when standing.

WEEK TWO CUE

Imagine that a horizontal shelf extends from your breastbone out into the space in front of you. Balance a glass on this shelf. Whenever you see a smile this week, check your posture and "balance the glass on the B-shelf".

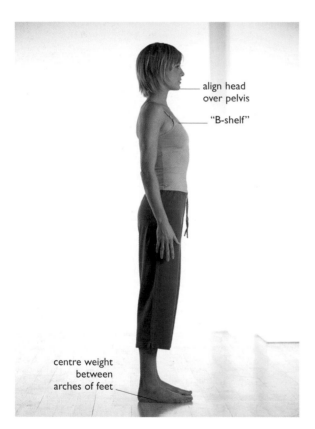

align head over pelvis

"B-shelf"

centre weight between arches of feet

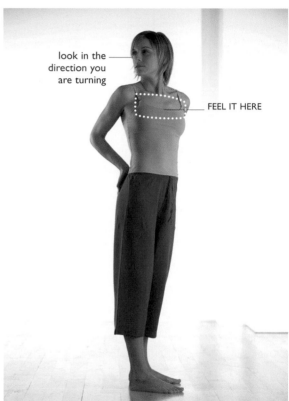

look in the direction you are turning

FEEL IT HERE

1 Stand with feet just less than hip-width apart. Check that your head is aligned over your pelvis. You may need to move your pelvis slightly forwards so that your centre of gravity falls in between the arches of your feet. Pull your navel into your spine, and lift the whole abdominal area from the pubis to the navel. Hold for 4 breath cycles, then relax.

2 Place your hands, fingers pointing down, on your lower back. Lift your chest up by balancing the imaginary glass on the "B-shelf". Turn your shoulders to the right, imagining that someone is pulling your right elbow behind you. Look to your right, turning your chin on the same level until you feel a comfortable stretch. Hold for 4 breath cycles, then repeat, turning to the left.

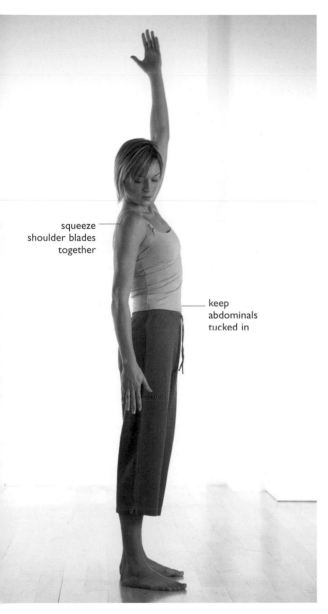

squeeze
shoulder blades
together

keep
abdominals
tucked in

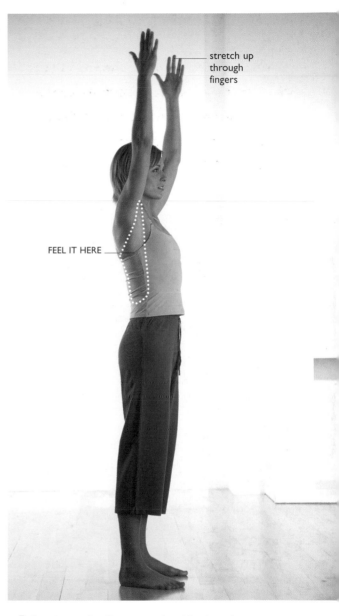

stretch up
through
fingers

FEEL IT HERE

3 Reach one arm up and the other down by your side. Turn your palms to face in, and imagine that someone is pulling the third fingers of each hand up and down respectively. As you reach up with your top hand, look down towards your bottom hand, pulling it down further. Hold for 4 breath cycles, then release. Repeat with the opposite arm raised.

4 Stand straight. Keep your head back against an imaginary wall. Lengthen and open your waist by lifting your ribcage. Reach both arms up as high as you comfortably can. Bring your shoulders down away from your ears, but keep the length of the waist. Imagine that someone is pulling the tips of your third fingers up towards the ceiling. Hold for 4 breath cycles, then relax.

WEEK THREE

In the final week of the programme, you perform a new set of stretches. Now the focus is mobility. Your posture should be erect but your body should be lithe. These deep stretches encourage more spine rotation and will also improve stride length. Pay attention to technique when performing this 15-minute routine.

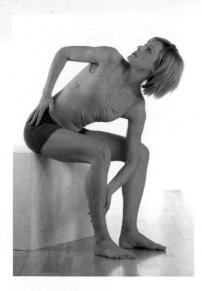

1 Sit slightly forwards on a chair, your feet flat on the floor. Lean forwards, hinging from your hips, and place your left elbow between your knees. Twist to the right, pulling your left shoulder downwards and pressing your left elbow against your left thigh to twist further. Feel the stretch under your arm, across your chest, and through your right hip. Hold for 4 breath cycles, then repeat on the other side.

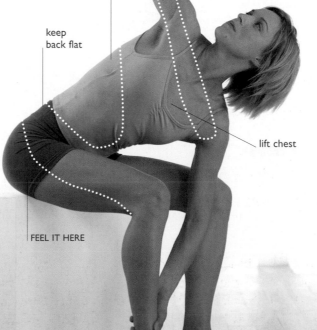

FEEL IT HERE

keep back flat

lift chest

FEEL IT HERE

2 Still seated, lean forwards and position your left upper arm between your knees. Hold on to your right ankle, and slowly reach your right hand up towards the ceiling. Turn your head and look up at your hand. Hold the stretch for 4 breath cycles, then repeat on the other side. Sit upright.

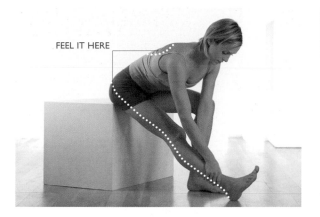

FEEL IT HERE

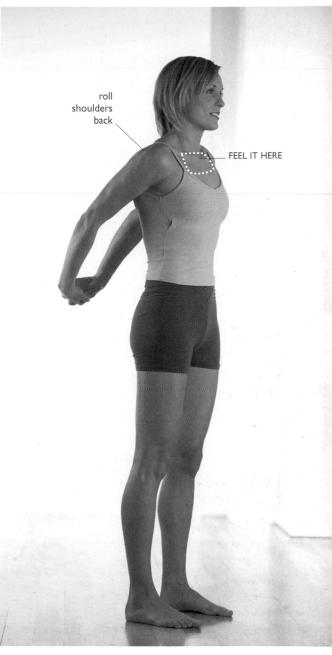

roll shoulders back

FEEL IT HERE

3 Place your right heel in front of you, straightening, or partially straightening, your leg. Lean forwards, flattening your back. Hold on to your shin or ankle, whichever is most comfortable. Stay for 4 breath cycles, then repeat on the other side. Return to sitting upright.

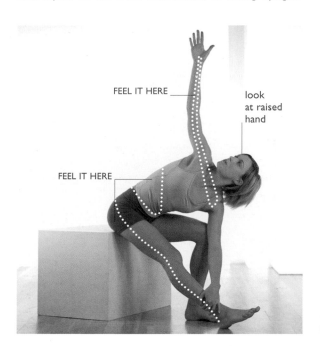

FEEL IT HERE

look at raised hand

FEEL IT HERE

4 Place your right heel in front of you again, with your leg straight. Lean forwards and grasp the shin or ankle of your right leg with your left hand. Reach up with your right hand, twisting as far as is comfortable. Hold for 4 breath cycles. Repeat on the other side.

5 Stand with feet just less than hip-width apart (as for the standing exercises in Week Two). Clasp your hands behind you and reach back as far as you can, taking care to keep your head aligned over your pelvis and your chin slightly tucked. Hold for 4 breath cycles.

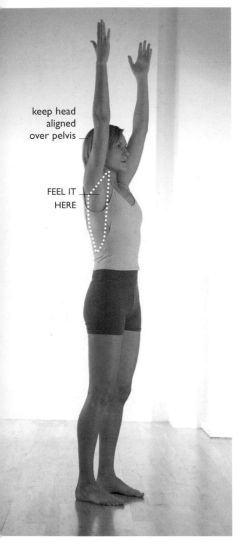

keep head
aligned
over pelvis

FEEL IT
HERE

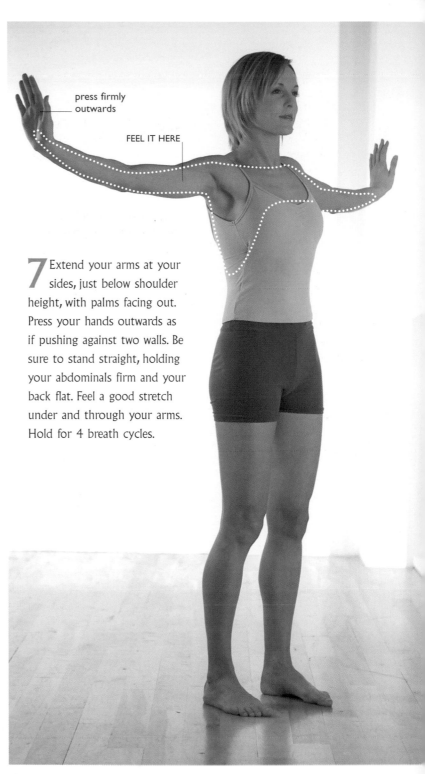

press firmly
outwards

FEEL IT HERE

7 Extend your arms at your sides, just below shoulder height, with palms facing out. Press your hands outwards as if pushing against two walls. Be sure to stand straight, holding your abdominals firm and your back flat. Feel a good stretch under and through your arms. Hold for 4 breath cycles.

6 With feet still positioned as for step 5, tuck your chin in slightly and align your head over your pelvis. Stretch both your arms up, bringing them as close to your head as possible while pulling your shoulders down. Feel the stretch in your armpits and through your shoulders. Hold for 4 breath cycles.

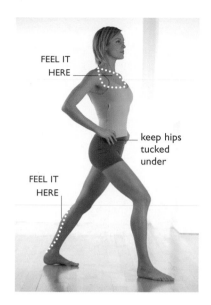

FEEL IT HERE

keep hips tucked under

FEEL IT HERE

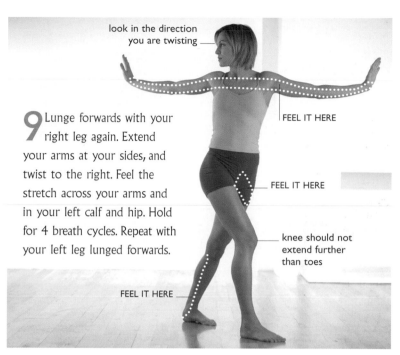

look in the direction you are twisting

FEEL IT HERE

FEEL IT HERE

knee should not extend further than toes

FEEL IT HERE

8 Step your right foot forwards into a lunge. Bend your right knee, but keep your left leg straight and your heel down. Place your hands on your hips, and press forwards. Hold for 4 breath cycles, then repeat on the other side. Step your feet back together again.

9 Lunge forwards with your right leg again. Extend your arms at your sides, and twist to the right. Feel the stretch across your arms and in your left calf and hip. Hold for 4 breath cycles. Repeat with your left leg lunged forwards.

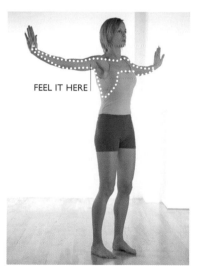

FEEL IT HERE

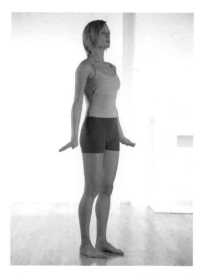

10 Step back so that your feet are hip-width apart, and align your head over your pelvis. Stand straight and press your palms outwards as in step 7. Hold for 4 breath cycles.

11 Lower your arms at your sides. Pull your fingers up as you press your hands down. At the same time, elongate your neck and stretch up through your head. Hold for 4 breath cycles, then relax.

PROGRAMME SUMMARY

It won't take you long to learn each week's simple stretches. Then use these quick-reference charts to remind you of the correct order in which to perform them. When you have completed the programme, you may find that you enjoy returning to a particular sequence. Remember to be conscientious about good technique. Breathe deeply and regularly throughout each sequence.

WEEK ONE

Be sure to keep your head aligned over your pelvis during these seated stretches, and perform them on both sides. Hold each position for 4 breath cycles.

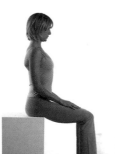

step 1 *p55*

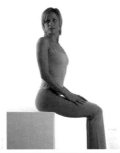

step 2 *p55*

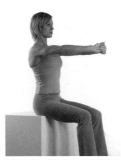

step 3 *p56*

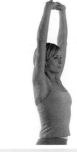

step 4 *p56*

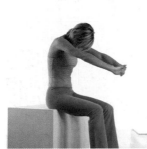

step 5 *p56*

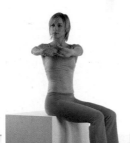

step 6 *p56*

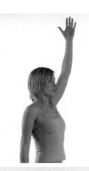

step 7 *p57*

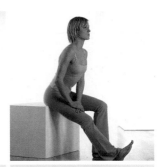

step 8 *p57*

WEEK TWO

Add these standing stretches to Week One's routine. Keep the head, spine, and pelvis aligned. Perform the stretches on both sides. Hold each position for 4 breath cycles.

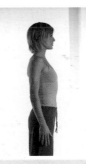

step 1 *p58*

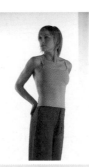

step 2 *p58*

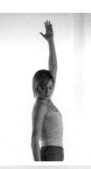

step 3 *p59*

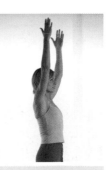

step 4 *p59*

WEEK THREE

With the focus now on mobility, these deep stretches improve general body flexibility. Perform the stretches on both sides, and hold each position for 4 breath cycles.

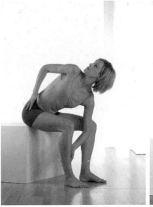

step 1 p60

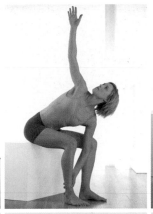

step 2 p60

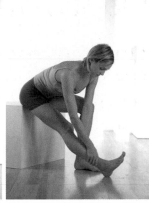

step 3 p61

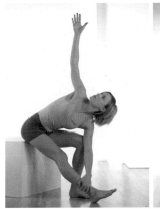

step 4 p61

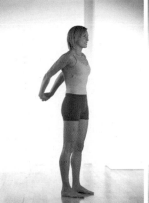

step 5 p61

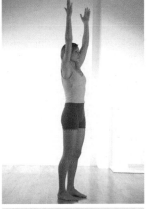

step 6 p62

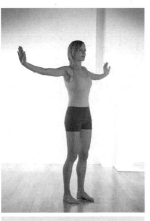

step 7 p62

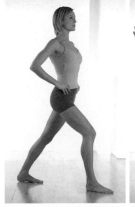

step 8 p63

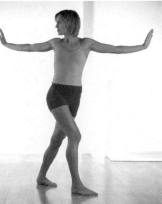

step 9 p63

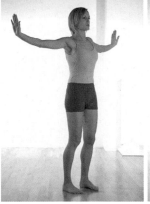

step 10 p63

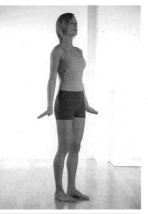

step 11 p63

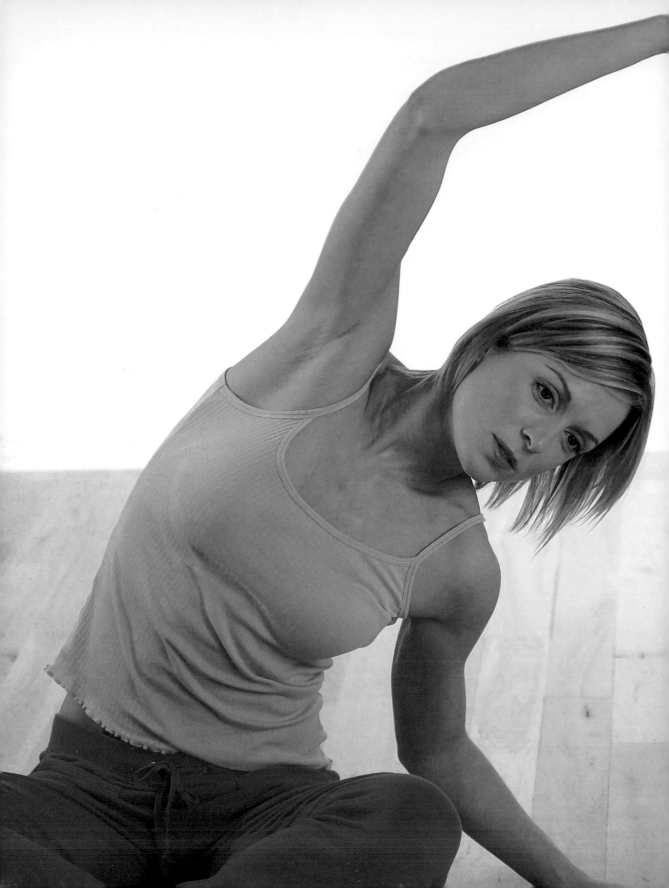

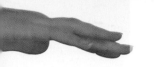

BASIC STRETCHING ROUTINES

Here I present three simple routines to help you incorporate stretching into your life. The Morning Wake-Up routine can be performed while still in bed and will centre and refresh you for the day ahead. The Relaxing Wind-Down routine will help to diffuse tension and prepare you for sleep. Try the Energizing Warm-Up to limber up before sports, or just as a revitalizing pick-me-up during the day. Make performing a stretching routine a habit and part of your daily ritual – discover what a difference it can make to your life.

MORNING WAKE-UP

We all need a little help getting our days started. Our joints tend to be stiff from lying in the same position all night, and our circulation sluggish. Begin slowly in the morning. Stretch gently, re-oxygenating the body and waking it up bit by bit. Use this five-minute routine to ease yourself out of bed and energize you for the day ahead.

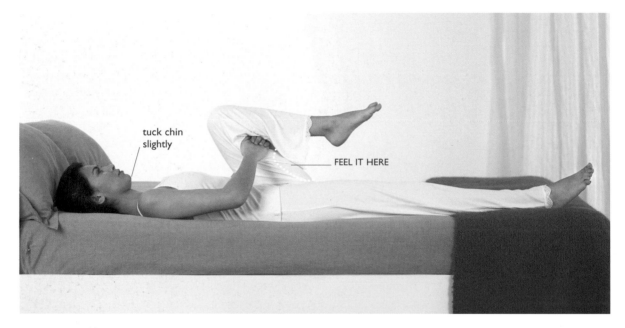

tuck chin slightly

FEEL IT HERE

1 Begin lying in bed on your back with your legs extended. Exhale and gently press your lower back into the mattress as you draw one knee towards your chest. Inhale, then exhale again as you pull your thigh closer into your chest. Then extend your leg, and repeat with the other leg.

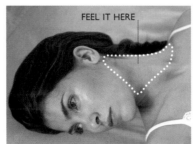

FEEL IT HERE

2 Tuck your chin in slightly. Exhale and slowly turn your head to the right. Inhale, then exhale and turn to the left. Repeat this 2 more times on each side.

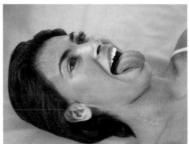

3 Open your eyes very wide, then blink 3 times. Now stick your tongue out, really stretching it, and say "ahhh" as you slowly exhale for a count of 4.

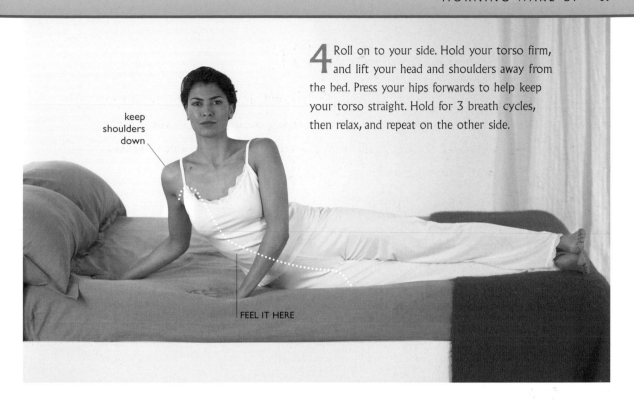

keep
shoulders
down

FEEL IT HERE

4 Roll on to your side. Hold your torso firm, and lift your head and shoulders away from the bed. Press your hips forwards to help keep your torso straight. Hold for 3 breath cycles, then relax, and repeat on the other side.

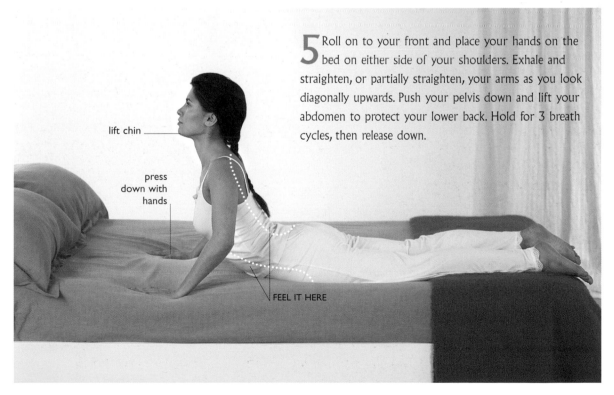

lift chin

press
down with
hands

FEEL IT HERE

5 Roll on to your front and place your hands on the bed on either side of your shoulders. Exhale and straighten, or partially straighten, your arms as you look diagonally upwards. Push your pelvis down and lift your abdomen to protect your lower back. Hold for 3 breath cycles, then release down.

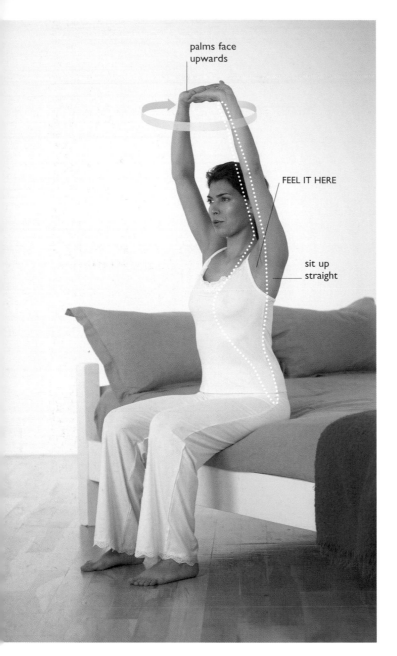

palms face
upwards

FEEL IT HERE

sit up
straight

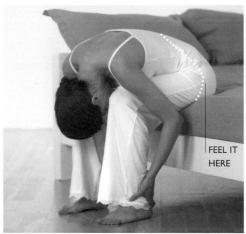

FEEL IT
HERE

7 Pull your abdominals into your spine as you lean forwards and grasp your ankles. Let your head hang. Feel this in your buttocks and lower back, and possibly in the backs of your legs and shins. Hold for 3 breath cycles.

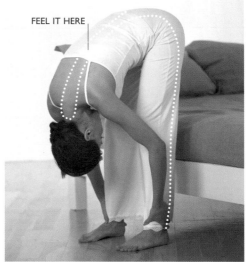

FEEL IT HERE

6 Sit on the edge of the bed with your feet on the floor. Clasp your hands with palms facing outwards. Exhale and tighten your abdominals as you reach your clasped hands up over your head. Breath consciously in and out as you circle 3 times in each direction. Then lower your hands.

8 Bring your hips off the bed so they are aligned over your feet in an upside-down stretch. Tighten your abdominals and lift your groin. Hold on to your ankles, nearby furniture, or the floor to help your balance. Keep your knees slightly bent. Hold for 2 breath cycles.

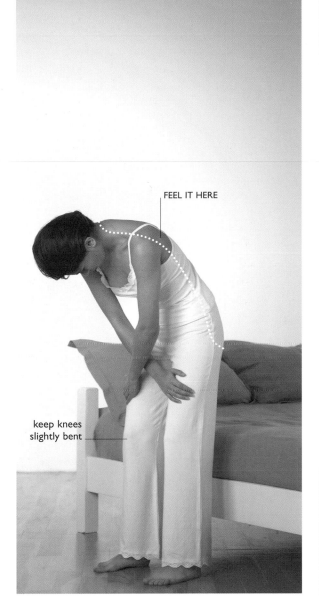

FEEL IT HERE

keep knees
slightly bent

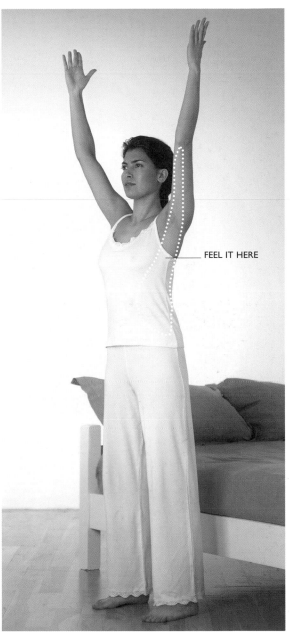

FEEL IT HERE

9 Slowly roll up. Feel your bottom anchoring your hips down towards the floor, and the heaviness of your head counterbalancing that anchor. As your hands reach thigh level, cross them and raise them above your head as if taking off an imaginary shirt.

10 Raise your hands above your head. Stretch up, feeling as if your third fingers and the tips of your ears are being pulled upwards. Take a deep breath in, then exhale and gently lower your hands while still standing up straight. Approach your day feeling centred and prepared.

RELAXING WIND-DOWN

Everyone needs a wind-down ritual at the end of the day. This routine prepares your body and mind for sleep by helping you to relax and to let go of the day's events. Consciously release tension as you perform these stretches, and feel stiff areas such as the overused chest and hips loosening up. Breathe slowly and regularly throughout. The routine should take approximately 10 minutes to complete.

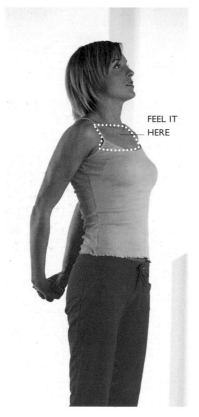

FEEL IT
HERE

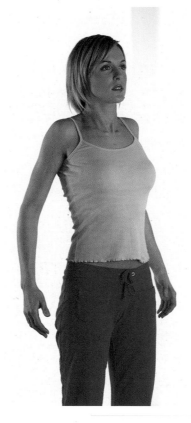

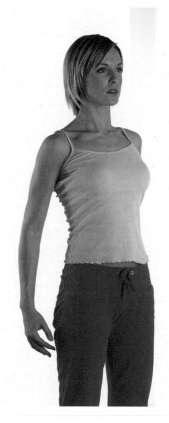

1 Tuck your hips under, and reach your clasped hands back behind you as far as they will comfortably go. Look diagonally upwards and hold for 3 breath cycles, opening your chest and arms. Release and bring your arms to your sides.

2 Keeping your hips tucked under, squeeze your shoulder blades together, pulling your shoulders back. Hold for 3 breath cycles, then release.

3 Stand up straight and pull your shoulders downwards. Focus the stretch by imagining that your little fingers and thumbs are being pulled towards the floor. Keep your head aligned over your spine. Hold for 3 breath cycles, then release.

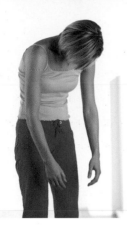

6 Intensify the stretch by moving your left arm to the inside of your thigh. Turn your chest to the right and reach your right arm up while pressing your left shoulder against your left thigh. Look at your right hand. Hold for 3 breath cycles, then release. Repeat steps 5 and 6 on the other side.

4 Tuck your chin into your chest and slowly round your shoulders forwards, hollowing your chest and caving it inwards. Keep your hips tucked under. Feel the stretch across your back. Hold for 3 breath cycles.

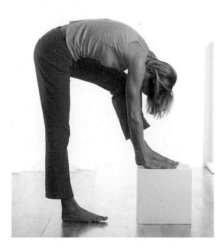

5 Place your left foot on the seat of a chair, knee bent. Pull your navel into your spine, bend forwards, and place your hands on either side of your raised foot to help your balance. Allow your head to hang down. Hold for 3 breath cycles.

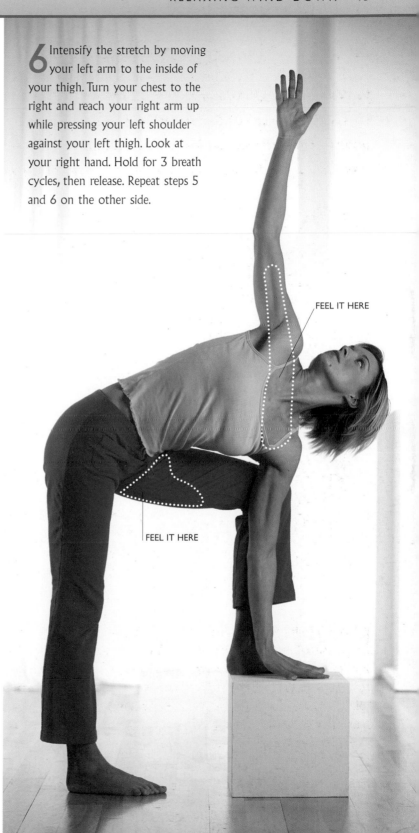

FEEL IT HERE

FEEL IT HERE

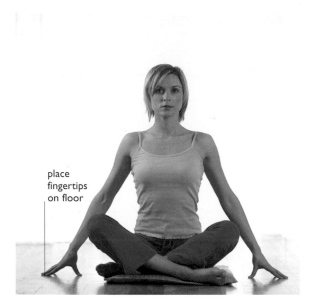

place
fingertips
on floor

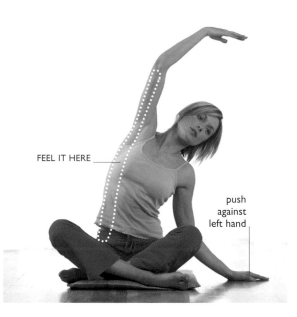

FEEL IT HERE

push
against
left hand

7 Sit on the floor with legs crossed. Use a cushion or folded towel to raise you up if your hips are too tight or your feet are uncomfortable. Sit up straight, and touch the floor on either side with your fingertips. This is your start position for sweeping semi-circle stretches.

8 Push your right hip into the floor as you reach your right arm up and to the left. Imagine that a big hook is pulling the side of your ribcage up to the ceiling. Place your left hand on the floor. Keep your back straight by imagining you are against a wall.

9 Sweep your arm down and across, letting your head and shoulders come forwards. Round forwards as if curving over a big beach ball. Place your hands, fingertips only, on the floor in front of you.

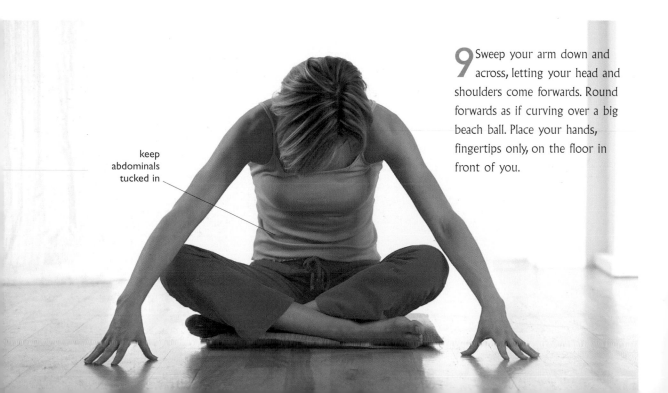

keep
abdominals
tucked in

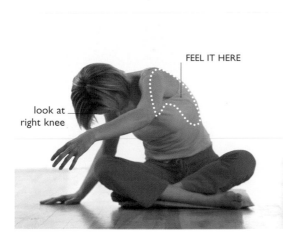

look at right knee

FEEL IT HERE

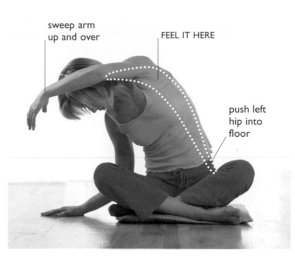

sweep arm up and over

FEEL IT HERE

push left hip into floor

10 Staying low, sweep your left arm across to the right in a smooth motion as you place your right hand on the floor and begin to push against it. Remember to keep your abdominals tight to help protect your lower back.

11 Sweep your left arm up as you push your left hip into the floor and lean to the right. Sweep your arm over, opening the chest, and return to the step 7 position. Then reverse the semi-circle: raise your left arm and sweep in the opposite direction. Repeat 3 times in each direction.

12 Finish by lying on your back with your calves supported on the seat of a chair. Position your knees in line over your hips. Cross your arms across your chest and take at least 6 slow, deep breaths in then out. As you inhale, imagine the mercury in a thermometer expanding from your tail to your head, then relax your body fully as you exhale.

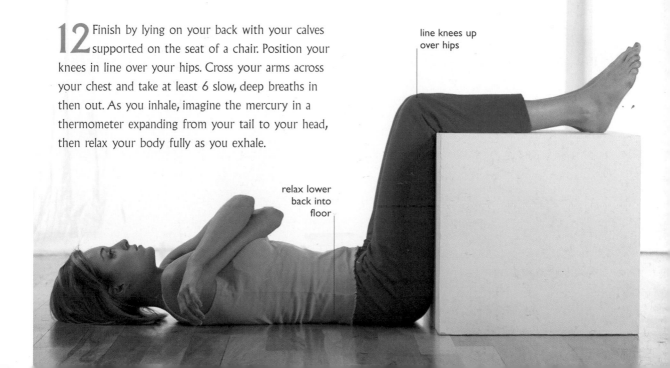

line knees up over hips

relax lower back into floor

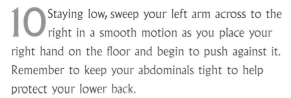

ENERGIZING WARM-UP

Before any physical activity, and especially before sports, it's important to limber up. This 5-minute sequence of moving stretches will increase mobility by lubricating the joints and increasing circulation to the muscles and tendons. You are in effect turning the muscles "on", improving reaction time and co-ordination, and preparing them to participate more fully in an activity or sport.

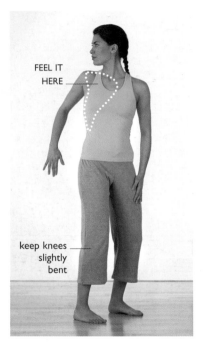

FEEL IT HERE

keep knees slightly bent

1 Stand with your feet slightly more than shoulder-width apart, arms at your sides. Pull your navel into your spine, and tuck your hips under. Roll your right shoulder forwards, up, back, then down. Then roll your left shoulder back in the same way. Repeat 10 times, alternating between shoulders. Allow your chin and chest to follow the movement of your shoulders.

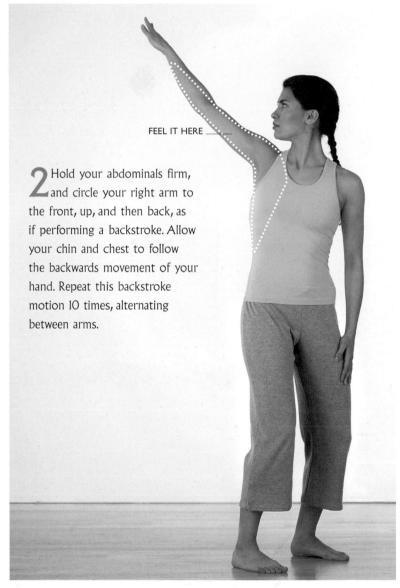

FEEL IT HERE

2 Hold your abdominals firm, and circle your right arm to the front, up, and then back, as if performing a backstroke. Allow your chin and chest to follow the backwards movement of your hand. Repeat this backstroke motion 10 times, alternating between arms.

3 Place your hands on your hips. Hold on to something for balance, if needed. Keep your back straight, and swing one leg straight up in front of you.

4 Then swing your leg down and back. Feel the weight of your leg come down with your foot and rotate the toes gently outwards. Repeat the swinging motion, steps 3 and 4, 10 times, then do the same with the other leg.

FEEL IT HERE

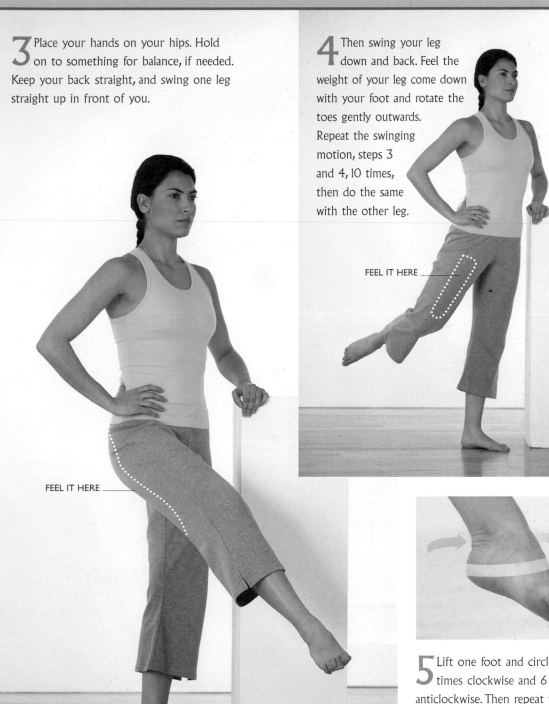

FEEL IT HERE

5 Lift one foot and circle it 6 times clockwise and 6 times anticlockwise. Then repeat with the other foot.

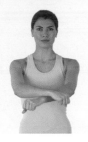 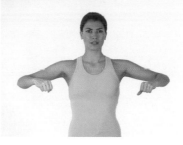 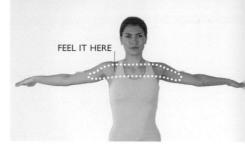

6 Stand with your feet shoulder-width apart, your hips tucked under. Bend both elbows and make loose fists with your hands. Raise your arms to shoulder height and cross them in front of your chest.

7 Pull your elbows out to the sides and press back to open your chest. Hold your torso steady and keep your arms bent. Then cross your elbows back in front of your chest as in step 6.

8 Gently swing your elbows back, opening your arms and throwing your hands back. Then bring your arms in and return to the step 6 start position with elbows crossed in front of your chest. Repeat steps 6–8, alternating this hook and swing motion, 6 times.

9 Keep your hips tucked under, and pull your navel into your spine. With elbows loose, swing your arms up and cross your wrists above your head.

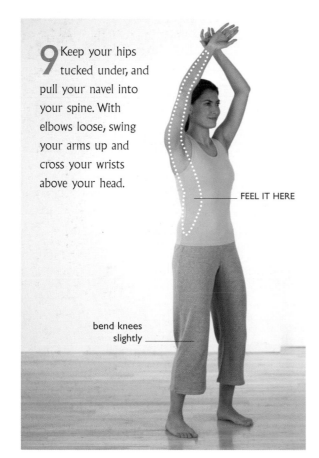

FEEL IT HERE

bend knees slightly

10 Swing your arms down and behind you. Repeat this alternating up-and-down swinging motion, steps 9 and 10, 6 times.

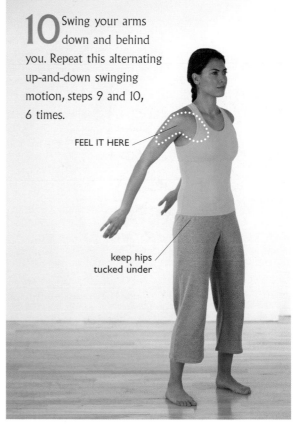

FEEL IT HERE

keep hips tucked under

11 Place your left hand on your hip and cross your right foot over your left. Tuck your hips under to help focus the stretch in the front of the IT band, the tendon that runs down the side of the hip and thigh. Stretch your right arm up, and lean into your left hip. Hold for 4 breath cycles. Repeat on the other side.

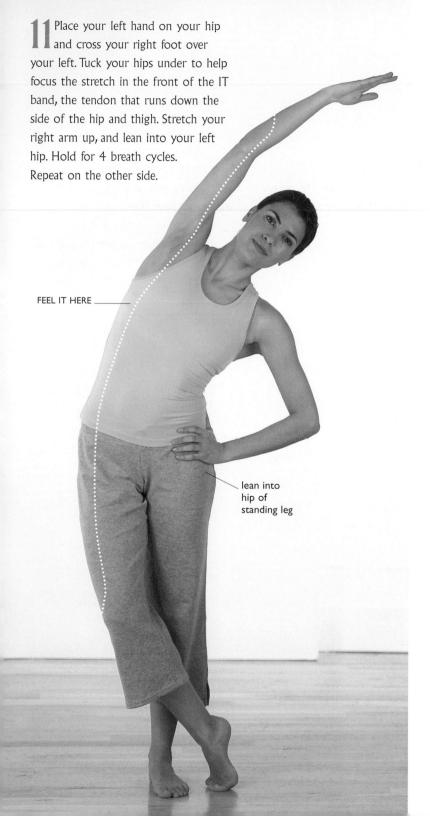

FEEL IT HERE

lean into hip of standing leg

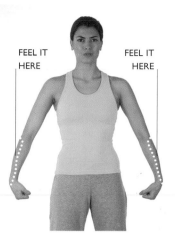

FEEL IT HERE

FEEL IT HERE

12 Stand straight with chest lifted and arms by your sides. Curl your fingers and wrists under as if trying to touch the insides of your forearms. Feel the stretch in your outer forearms and hold for a count of 3, then release.

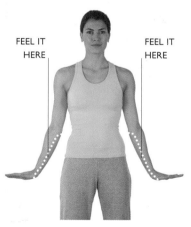

FEEL IT HERE

FEEL IT HERE

13 Curl your fingers and wrists up, feeling the stretch in your inner forearms. Hold for a count of 3, then release. Alternate between steps 12 and 13, curling your fingers under and up 6 times.

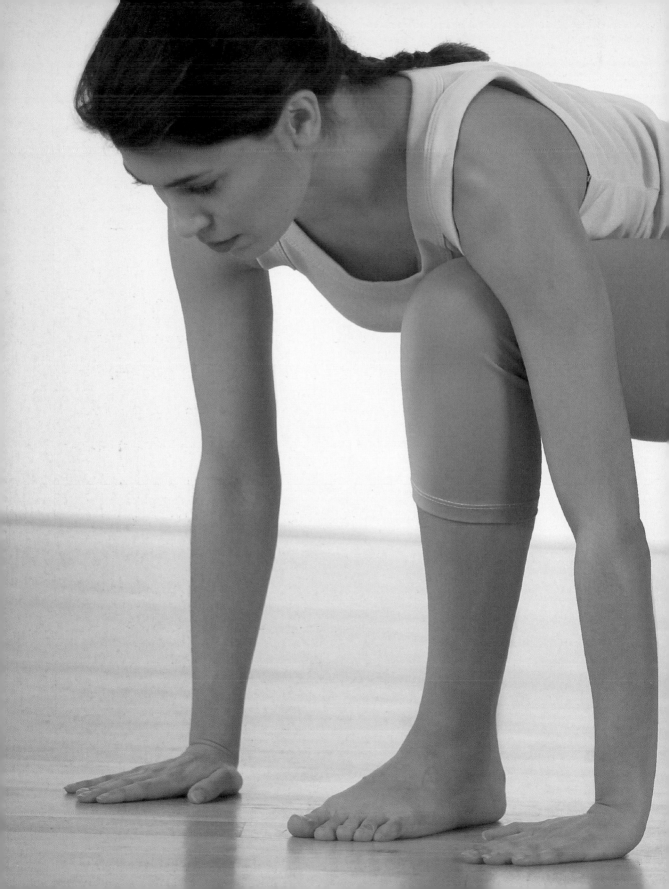

STRETCHES FOR SPORTS

Stretching before sports helps to prepare the muscles for action and for moving into more strenuous positions than everyday life. After sports, it helps the tissues to relax and enables exercise by-products, which cause muscle soreness, to circulate out of the bloodstream. The stretches in the pages that follow will help you to meet the demands of each particular sport. Be sure to limber up with the Energizing Warm-up (see pp.76–79) before sports, then add on these extra stretches before and after your session. Whether you are swimming, cycling, or playing tennis, let the stretches presented here serve as your tailor-made sports routines.

TENNIS

The stretches here focus on the muscles of the upper body. Gripping the racket and performing the large movements of the forearm and backhand strokes can place great demands on the shoulders, arms, and hands. If possible, add the Outer Thigh Stretch (*see p.45*) to your routine to help knee health.

FOREARM EXTENSOR

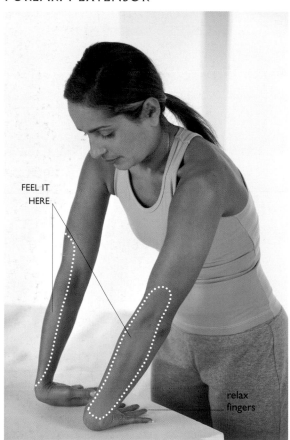

Place your hands, knuckles down and fingers pointing towards you, on a surface in front of you. Lean your weight forwards slightly, and roll with pressure towards your wrists. Lean back to increase the stretch along the fronts of your forearms. Hold for 3 breath cycles.

FOREARM FLEXOR

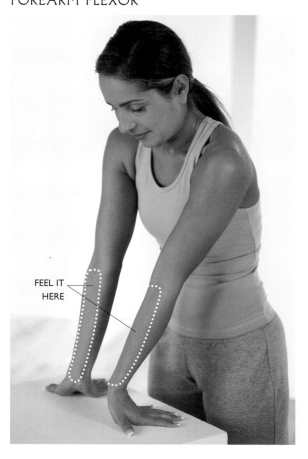

Place your hands, palms down with fingers splayed and pointing towards you, on a surface in front of you. Gently lean forwards on to your palms, then pull back with your body to increase the stretch along the insides of your forearms. Hold for 3 breath cycles.

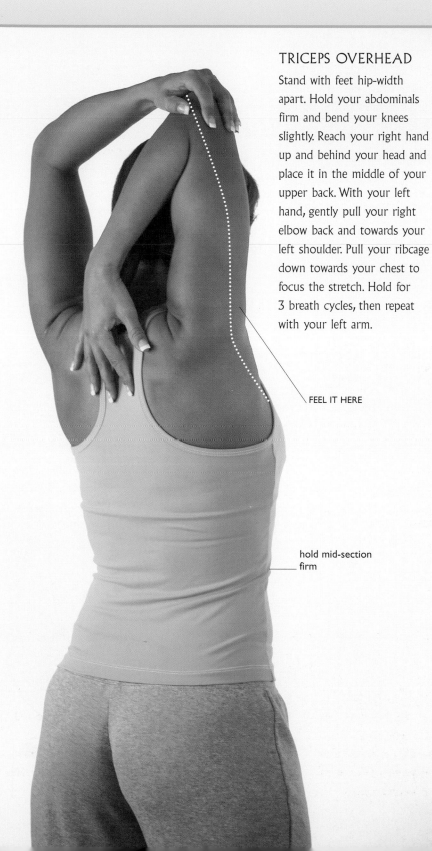

TRICEPS OVERHEAD

Stand with feet hip-width apart. Hold your abdominals firm and bend your knees slightly. Reach your right hand up and behind your head and place it in the middle of your upper back. With your left hand, gently pull your right elbow back and towards your left shoulder. Pull your ribcage down towards your chest to focus the stretch. Hold for 3 breath cycles, then repeat with your left arm.

FEEL IT HERE

hold mid-section firm

MINI CATALOGUE

These stretches focus on the hands, arms, chest, and ribcage. Flexibility and strength in these areas will help to improve your game.

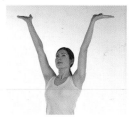

arms open *p29*
hold for 3 breath cycles

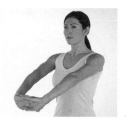

arm stretch *p28*
hold for 3 breath cycles

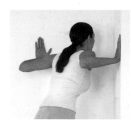

corner chest stretch *p30*
hold for 4 breath cycles

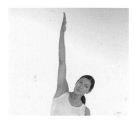

standing side stretch *p31*
hold for 4 breath cycles;
repeat on other side

GOLF

The motion of swinging a golf club involves twisting the spine, shoulders, and hips. Golfers also need to be able to shift their weight sideways from one leg to the other while keeping their feet on the ground. Stretching will improve your swing and protect your back. Be sure to include the Side Hip Stretch (*see opposite*).

STRETCHING HELPS TO:
• **increase power** behind a swing by enabling better wind-up through increased back mobility.
• **improve follow-through** after a swing by increasing hip and shoulder mobility.

CROSSED ARMS TWIST

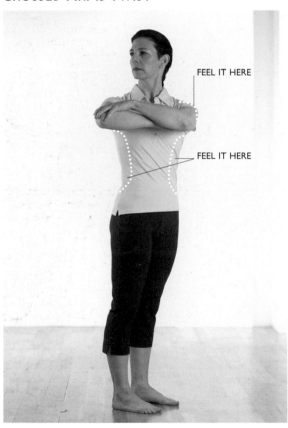

FEEL IT HERE

FEEL IT HERE

OVERHEAD CROSSED ARMS TWIST

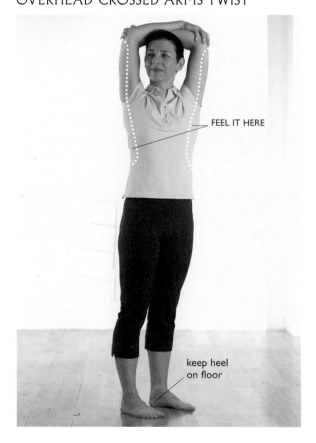

FEEL IT HERE

keep heel on floor

Stand with feet hip-width apart. Squeeze your buttocks to anchor your lower body. Clasp your elbows and raise them to shoulder height. Twist your shoulders and upper body to the right. Gently pull your left elbow with your right hand, and look to the right. Hold for 4 breath cycles. Repeat, twisting to the left.

Stand with feet hip-width apart and chest lifted. Squeeze your buttocks to anchor your lower body. Reach your arms upwards, holding the bottom of your ribcage down. Twist your upper body to the right. Keep your shoulders down and away from your ears, and hold for 3 breath cycles. Repeat, twisting to the left.

BACKWARDS WRIST PULL

Stand with feet hip-width apart. Squeeze your buttocks to anchor your lower body. Roll your shoulders up and back, and grasp your left wrist behind you. Hold the bottom of your ribcage down as you lift your chest. Twist to the left, gently pulling your wrist to the right behind you. Hold for 3 breath cycles; repeat on the other side.

turn head in direction of twist

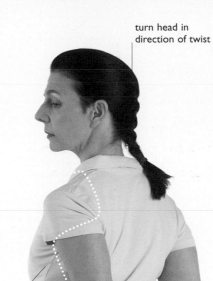

FEEL IT HERE

MINI CATALOGUE

Include this hand stretch to keep your grip strong yet precise, and add these torso and hip stretches to improve your swing.

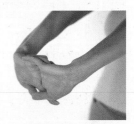

clasped fingers *p28*
hold for 3 breath cycles

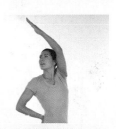

standing waist twist *p40*
hold for 2 breath cycles; repeat on other side

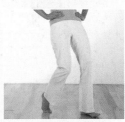

front hip stretch *p42*
hold for 3 breath cycles; repeat on other side

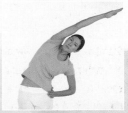

side hip stretch *p43*
hold for 4 breath cycles; repeat on other side

SWIMMING

A daily upper body stretching routine is essential for swimmers. The front crawl in particular involves tremendous repetitive shoulder work, which can tighten the head, neck, and shoulder muscles. This can cause not only shoulder joint problems, but also nerve pinches and general muscle stiffness.

STRETCHING HELPS TO:

- **make front crawl breathing** easier by increasing the flexibility of your neck.
- **improve your stroke length** by loosening and rebalancing overworked shoulders.

EAR-TO-SHOULDER NECK STRETCH

Stand straight, lift your chest, and pull your navel into your spine. Reach your right hand behind you and grasp your left arm just above the elbow. Tuck your chin into your chest. Let your right ear drop towards your right shoulder as you gently pull your left arm down. Focus on the area from the tip of the shoulder to the ear, breathing into the stretch. Hold for 3 breath cycles, then repeat on the other side.

FEEL IT HERE

grasp arm above elbow

keep buttocks firm

UPPER BACK SIDE-BEND AND TWIST

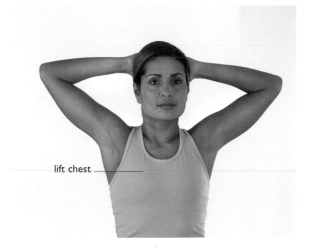

lift chest

1 Stand straight, and pull your navel into your spine. Clasp your hands behind your head. Gently press your head back, open your elbows, and lift your chest.

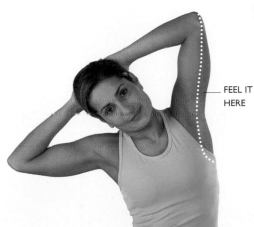

FEEL IT HERE

2 Slowly tilt your body to the right by raising your left elbow so that it points upwards. Inhale and exhale, feeling the stretch along your left arm. Don't allow your raised elbow to tilt forwards.

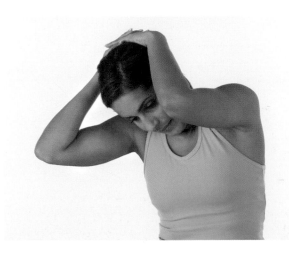

3 Still leaning to the right, lower your left elbow so that both elbows point downwards. Curve your chest as if rounding it over a ball. Inhale and exhale, feeling the stretch across your upper back. Then open your elbows and lift back up to vertical. Repeat on the other side.

MINI CATALOGUE

If you swim regularly, stay flexible by including these upper body and hand exercises in your stretching routine.

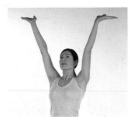

arms open *p29*
hold for 3 breath cycles

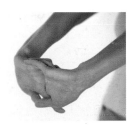

clasped fingers *p28*
hold for 3 breath cycles

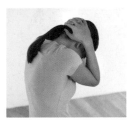

upper back forward stretch *p32*
hold for 2 breath cycles

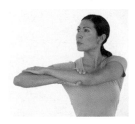

twist, arms crossed *p33*
hold for 2 breath cycles; repeat on other side

FOOTBALL

Football players need quick reactions and agility Running, stopping, starting, and kicking the ball involve moving your legs in many different planes, which requires good hip flexibility. These stretches will help prevent groin strains and counteract muscle tightness in the hips that can result from lots of running.

STRETCHING HELPS TO:

- **make running easier** by releasing tight hip and leg muscles and improving stride length.
- **make quick changes** of direction when running easier by improving back flexibility.

CURVE AND ARCH

The key to this stretch is to press your head back into your hands as you arch back.

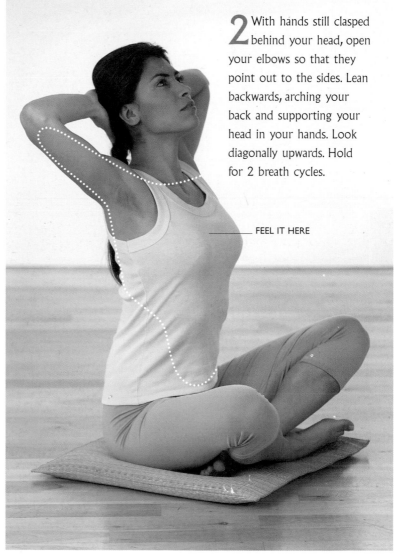

2 With hands still clasped behind your head, open your elbows so that they point out to the sides. Lean backwards, arching your back and supporting your head in your hands. Look diagonally upwards. Hold for 2 breath cycles.

FEEL IT HERE

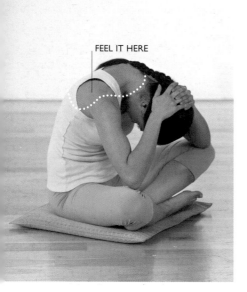

FEEL IT HERE

1 Sit up straight with your legs crossed. Lift your head and clasp your hands behind it. Point your elbows forwards. Tuck your chin in, and slowly roll your head down until your elbows touch your knees. Inhale and exhale, then slowly roll back up.

SITTING GROIN STRETCH

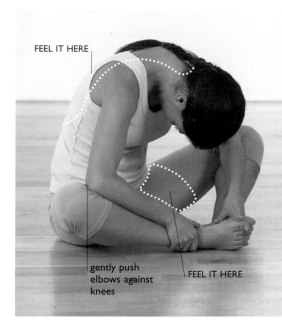

FEEL IT HERE

gently push elbows against knees

FEEL IT HERE

Sit on the floor with the soles of your feet together and your knees apart, falling towards the floor. Pull your navel into your spine, and gently hold on to your shins as you pull your head towards your feet. Gently pull your ankles to increase the stretch in the groin, back, and outer hips. Hold for 3–4 breath cycles.

LEANING HURDLER

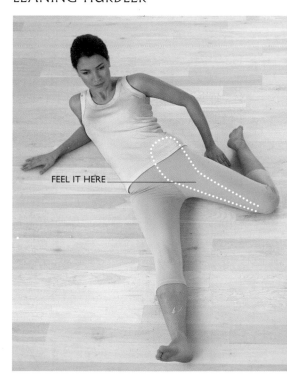

FEEL IT HERE

Avoid this stretch if you have knee problems. Sit on the floor and lean back, supporting yourself with your arms to prevent any strain on the knees. Bend your left leg, bringing your foot towards your bottom. Push your left hip forwards and pull your navel into your spine. Lean on your right forearm or hand and feel the stretch in the front of your hip and thigh. Hold for 3–4 breath cycles. Repeat on the other side.

MINI CATALOGUE

Be sure to include these lower body stretches. The hips, thighs, and calves become tight and fatigued from constant running.

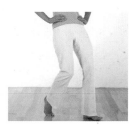

front hip stretch *p42*
hold for 3 breath cycles; repeat on other side

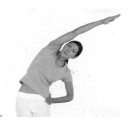

side hip stretch *p43*
hold for 4 breath cycles; repeat on other side

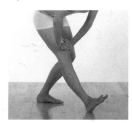

standing hamstring *p46*
hold for 3 breath cycles; repeat on other leg

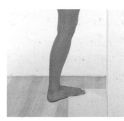

step drop *p49*
hold for 4 breath cycles

RUNNING

The nemesis of all runners is IT band friction syndrome, where the tendon that runs down the outside of the thigh becomes inflamed. Another common complaint is the dreaded piriformis syndrome, where the sciatic nerve becomes irritated and causes leg pain. These stretches will help to keep you running pain-free.

RUNNER'S LUNGE

Stretch your legs and hips to help balance your stride. Ensure that the "headlights" of your hips face forwards equally. Resist the tendency to twist to the right by pressing your right hip down towards the floor.

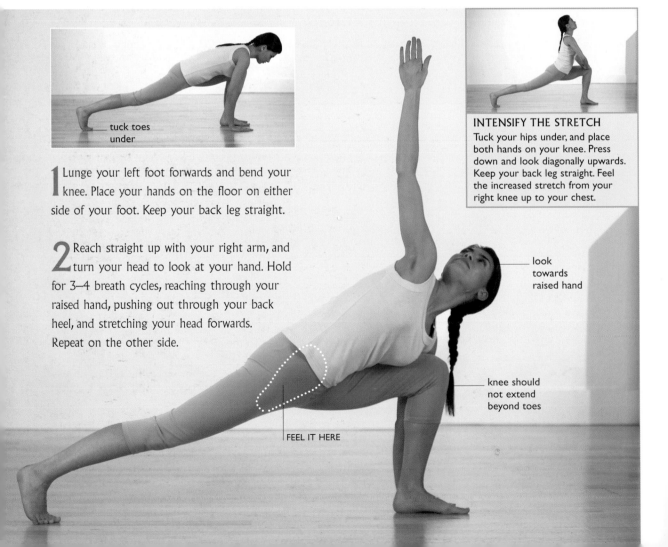

tuck toes under

1 Lunge your left foot forwards and bend your knee. Place your hands on the floor on either side of your foot. Keep your back leg straight.

2 Reach straight up with your right arm, and turn your head to look at your hand. Hold for 3–4 breath cycles, reaching through your raised hand, pushing out through your back heel, and stretching your head forwards. Repeat on the other side.

INTENSIFY THE STRETCH
Tuck your hips under, and place both hands on your knee. Press down and look diagonally upwards. Keep your back leg straight. Feel the increased stretch from your right knee up to your chest.

look towards raised hand

knee should not extend beyond toes

FEEL IT HERE

SEATED PIRIFORMIS TWIST

The piriformis muscle is behind the gluteal (buttock) muscle, close to the sciatic nerve. This stretch lengthens the muscles and helps preserve the nerve.

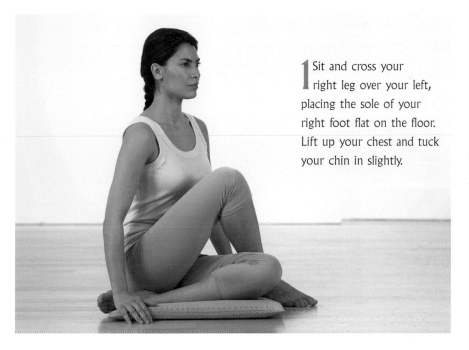

1 Sit and cross your right leg over your left, placing the sole of your right foot flat on the floor. Lift up your chest and tuck your chin in slightly.

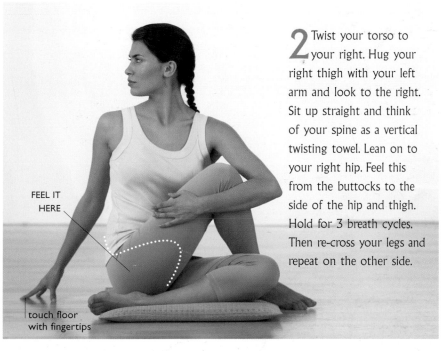

FEEL IT HERE

touch floor with fingertips

2 Twist your torso to your right. Hug your right thigh with your left arm and look to the right. Sit up straight and think of your spine as a vertical twisting towel. Lean on to your right hip. Feel this from the buttocks to the side of the hip and thigh. Hold for 3 breath cycles. Then re-cross your legs and repeat on the other side.

MINI CATALOGUE

These hip, leg, and foot stretches will have a restorative effect. Ensure that you are ready for your next run!

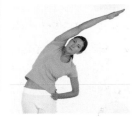

side hip stretch *p43*
hold for 4 breath cycles; repeat on other side

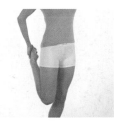

standing quad stretch *p44*
hold for 3 breath cycles; repeat on other leg

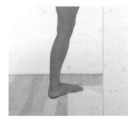

step drop *p49*
hold for 4 breath cycles

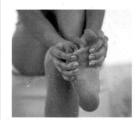

transverse arch *p51*
repeat both steps 5 times on each foot

SKIING

Whether cross-country or downhill, skiing uses the psoas muscles (the deep hip flexors), which run along either side of the spine and into the legs. Failing to stretch these muscles can cause lower back pain. It's also important to stretch the triceps, the muscles at the backs of the upper arms, which you use to handle ski poles.

> **STRETCHING HELPS TO:**
>
> • **improve balance and control** when skiing by developing an even squat stance.
>
> • **encourage good posture** and technique when skiing by helping to align the back.

PSOAS LUNGE

Remember to tuck your pelvis under when performing this stretch. Think of an imaginary tail attached to your tailbone – tuck your tail between your legs to tilt your pelvis under.

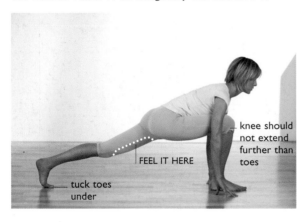

knee should not extend further than toes

FEEL IT HERE

tuck toes under

1 Lunge your right leg forwards, and place your hands on either side of your right foot. Straighten your back leg, and press your left hip towards the ground.

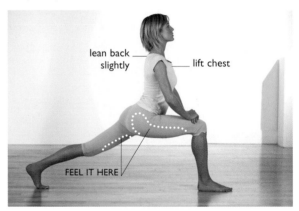

lean back slightly

lift chest

FEEL IT HERE

2 Tuck your hips under; place both hands on your right thigh. Exhale, lift your chest, and look diagonally upwards. Inhale, then exhale and look forwards.

3 Minding your balance, place your left forearm on your right thigh and slowly reach your right arm behind you. Then reach your left arm out so that both arms are extended. Look back in the direction of the twist and hold for 3 breath cycles. Repeat with your left leg lunged forwards.

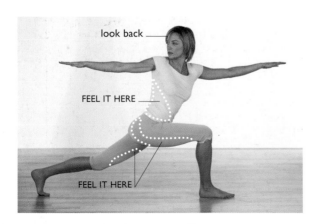

look back

FEEL IT HERE

FEEL IT HERE

LEANING TRICEPS STRETCH

Stand with feet about hip-width apart and pelvis tucked under. Cross your arms and hold on to your elbows. Lift upwards out of your waist and pull up with your hands as you lean up and over an imaginary fence on your left. Breathe into the stretch on your right side for 2 breath cycles, then return to upright and repeat on the other side.

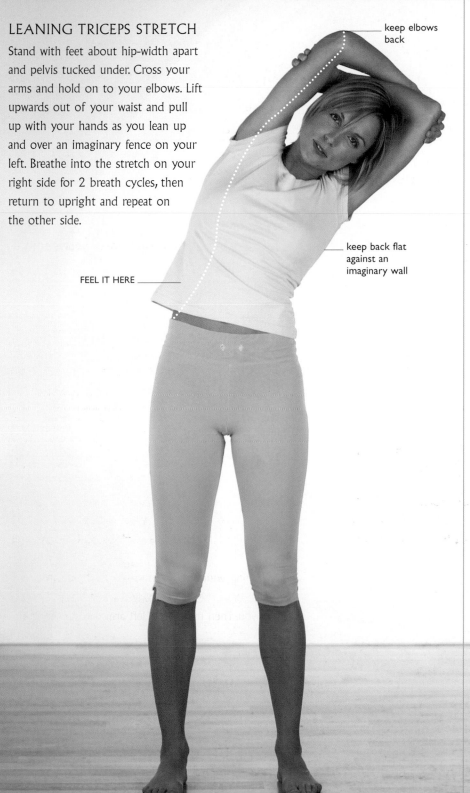

keep elbows back

keep back flat against an imaginary wall

FEEL IT HERE _____

MINI CATALOGUE

Skiing requires strong and flexible legs. Improve your stamina on the slopes by performing these simple hip and leg stretches.

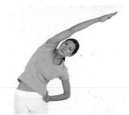

side hip stretch *p43*
hold for 4 breath cycles; repeat on other side

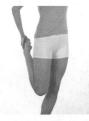

standing quad stretch *p44*
hold for 3 breath cycles; repeat on other leg

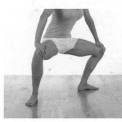

inner thigh squat *p45*
hold for 3 breath cycles

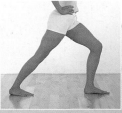

basic lunge *p48*
hold for 4 breath cycles; repeat on other leg

CYCLING

Regular cycling can cause tightness in the sides of the hips and the fronts of the thighs, leading to knee and back problems. The typical forwards-bent position may cause round shoulders, while tilting the head up to see ahead can pinch the neck nerves. Stretching helps to prevent these problems from being carried into daily life.

STRETCHING HELPS TO:

- **improve flexibility** for easier back and neck positioning over handle bars and frame.
- **restore and rebalance** over-used leg muscles, enabling greater power when cycling.

ANKLE-HOLD HIP STRETCH

This stretch targets the sides of the hips and the thighs – typical problem areas for cyclists.

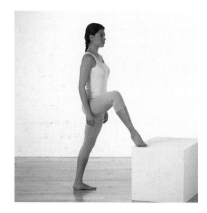

1 Hold your buttocks firm, then raise your right foot and place it on a stable support in front of you with knee bent. Raise your right heel so that just the ball of your foot is on the support.

2 Stretch up, pulling your ribs away from your pelvis, and lean forwards over your bent leg. Pull your navel into your spine, round your back, and grasp your ankle. Hold for 3 breath cycles, then repeat on the other leg.

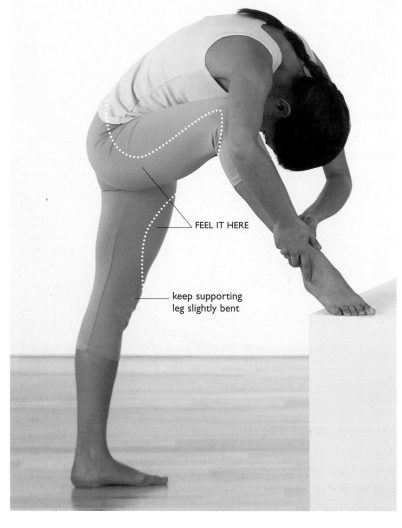

FEEL IT HERE

keep supporting leg slightly bent

SITTING, KNEES CROSSED

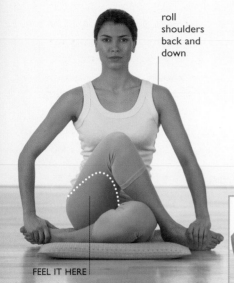

roll shoulders back and down

FEEL IT HERE

Sit on the floor with one leg crossed over the other, knees lined up, if possible. You may find it more comfortable to sit on a cushion or folded towel. Grasp your feet, and pull your navel in towards your spine. Pull your feet in towards you. Feel the stretch in the inner thighs and the sides of the hips. Hold for 3 breath cycles, then repeat with legs crossed the other way.

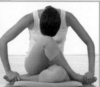

INTENSIFY THE STRETCH
Hold on to your feet and lean forwards as you pull your feet upwards. Feel an increased stretch in your thighs, hips, and upper back.

ELBOW GRASP

This is an excellent stretch to open the chest and shoulders. Grasp one arm and then the other. If you can't reach your elbows, hold your forearms.

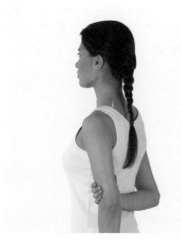

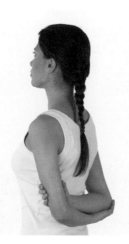

1 Stand with feet shoulder-width apart, your hips tucked under. Roll your shoulders up and back, pulling your shoulder blades together. Reach back and grasp your left arm above the elbow.

2 Then reach back and cup your right elbow in your left hand. Lift your chest, feeling the stretch there, and hold for 3 breath cycles. Re-cross your arms and repeat the stretch.

MINI CATALOGUE

These stretches will help to open the chest and stretch the waist. The leg stretches will combat tightness in the thighs.

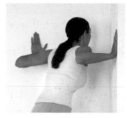

corner chest stretch *p30*
hold for 4 breath cycles

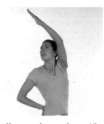

standing waist twist *p40*
hold for 2 breath cycles;
repeat on other side

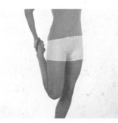

standing quad stretch *p44*
hold for 3 breath cycles;
repeat on other leg

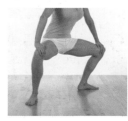

inner thigh squat *p45*
hold for 3 breath cycles

HIKING

An excellent sport for experiencing nature, hiking strengthens the lower back. The downside is that walking for long distances can cause tightness in the hips and legs. Wearing a backpack when you hike can strain the trapezius muscles between the neck and shoulders as they tense to push up against the extra weight.

STRETCHING HELPS TO:

- **increase stamina** for distance hiking by relaxing overused muscles in the hips and legs.
- **lessen soreness** and restore muscle length, increasing the overall enjoyment of hiking.

BOWED-HEAD KNEE HUG

Keep this stretch focused in the buttocks and back of the thigh by pressing your hips downwards as you lift your knee. Pulling your knee up towards the opposite shoulder in the second step intensifies this stretch.

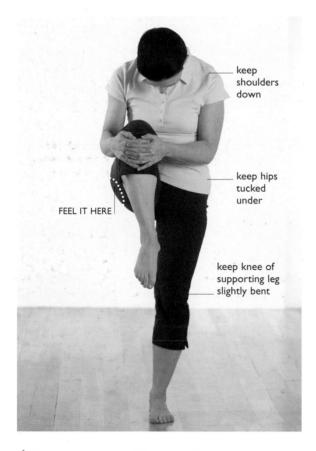

keep shoulders down

keep hips tucked under

FEEL IT HERE

keep knee of supporting leg slightly bent

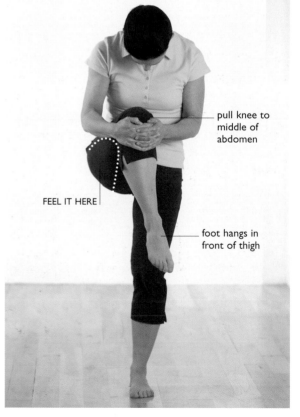

pull knee to middle of abdomen

FEEL IT HERE

foot hangs in front of thigh

1 Balance on one leg while you pull your other knee towards your chest. Tuck your hips under and bow your head towards your knee for 3 breath cycles.

2 Look forwards, then hug your raised knee towards the opposite shoulder. Bow your head again, and hold for 3 breath cycles. Repeat with the other leg.

HAND-ON-HEAD NECK STRETCH

This stretches the upper trapezius, which is responsible for elevating the shoulders, tilting the head to the same side, and rotating the chin towards the ceiling.

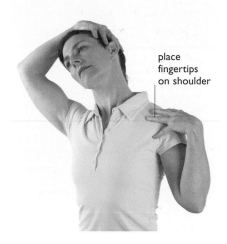

place fingertips on shoulder

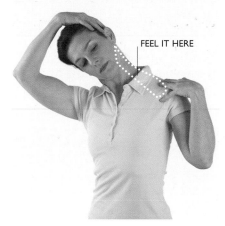

FEEL IT HERE

1 Place your left hand on your left shoulder and your right hand on your head, just above your left ear. Gently allow your right arm weight to pull your head towards your right shoulder.

2 Maintaining the gentle stretch in the left side of your neck, slowly turn your chin towards your left shoulder. Hold for 3 breath cycles, then repeat on the other side.

FRONT OF SHIN STRETCH

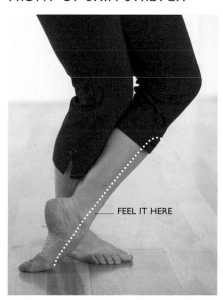

FEEL IT HERE

Cross your left leg in front of your right and point your left foot, placing it top-side down on the floor. Gently bend your right leg so that it presses down on your left calf. Feel the stretch in the front of your left shin and down into the front of the foot. Hold for 3 breath cycles. Repeat on the other foot.

MINI CATALOGUE

These stretches target the hips and thighs, which are in constant use when hiking. Be sure to stop for regular stretching breaks.

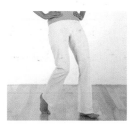

front hip stretch *p42*
hold for 3 breath cycles; repeat on other side

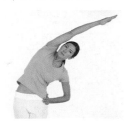

side hip stretch *p43*
hold for 4 breath cycles; repeat on other side

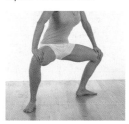

inner thigh squat *p45*
hold for 3 breath cycles

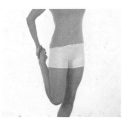

standing quad stretch *p44*
hold for 3 breath cycles; repeat on other leg

DANCING

A typical dance session may involve demanding footwork as well as some arm endurance from holding and changing arm positions. Dancers often develop problems with the IT bands – the tendons that run down the outsides of the thighs. When they become tight they can cause lower back soreness and aching legs.

STRETCHING HELPS TO:

- **make you lighter** on your feet by improving hip mobility and weight-shifting ability.
- **improve smoothness**, grace, and poise by enabling greater freedom of movement.

SEATED FIGURE 4

Feel this IT band stretch by lifting the ankle upwards as you press the knee downwards. There should be no pain in your knees. If you can't bring your ankle to your knee, cross your legs as comfortably as possible.

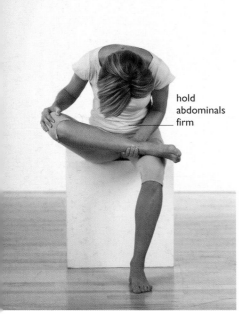

hold abdominals firm

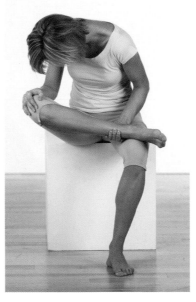

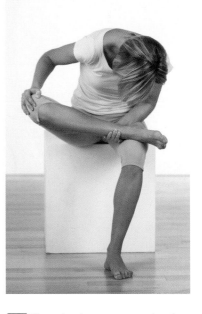

1 Sit slightly forwards on a chair. Cross your right leg over your left, slip your left hand under your crossed ankle, and place your right hand on your knee. Lean forwards from your hips as you gently pull your left ankle and bow your head down. Hold for 3 breath cycles.

2 Slowly move your head and upper body to the right so that you are looking at your knee. Keep your abdominals firm. Feel the stretch in the side of your right hip and hold for 3 breath cycles.

3 Then slowly move your head and upper body to the left so that you are looking at your foot. Feel the stretch at the bottom of your right hip. Hold for 3 breath cycles. Re-cross your legs and repeat the sequence of stretches on the other side.

STANDING HAND CLASP

1 Stand with your feet about shoulder-width apart, and tuck your pelvis under. Lift your kneecaps to straighten your legs and ensure that you don't press back into your knees. Clasp your hands behind your back.

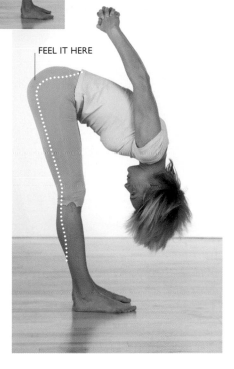

FEEL IT HERE

2 Roll your shoulders back, then lift your hands behind you. Pull your navel into your spine as you lean forwards. Squeeze your upper arms together as you raise your hands to a comfortable position. Feel a good stretch in your legs, but also in your arms and shoulders. Hold for 3 breath cycles.

STANDING WIND-UP

Stand with feet shoulder-width apart. Reach your arms around to the right, placing your hands on your hips. Wind yourself up tightly as you turn your head and look around to the right. Feel a good stretch in your back and some stretch in your shoulders and waist. Hold for 3 breath cycles; repeat on the other side.

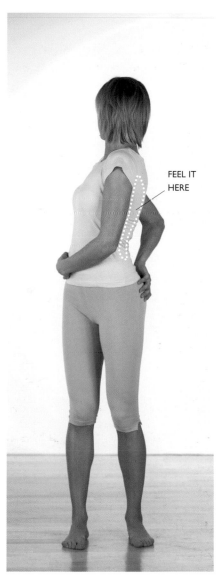

FEEL IT HERE

MINI CATALOGUE

Be sure to perform these simple hip and leg stretches before and after any recreational dance session.

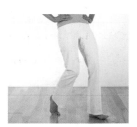

front hip stretch *p42*
hold for 3 breath cycles; repeat on other side

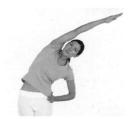

side hip stretch *p43*
hold for 4 breath cycles; repeat on other side

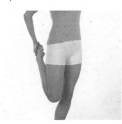

standing quad stretch *p44*
hold for 3 breath cycles repeat on other leg

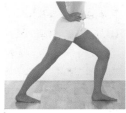

basic lunge *p48*
hold for 4 breath cycles; repeat on other leg

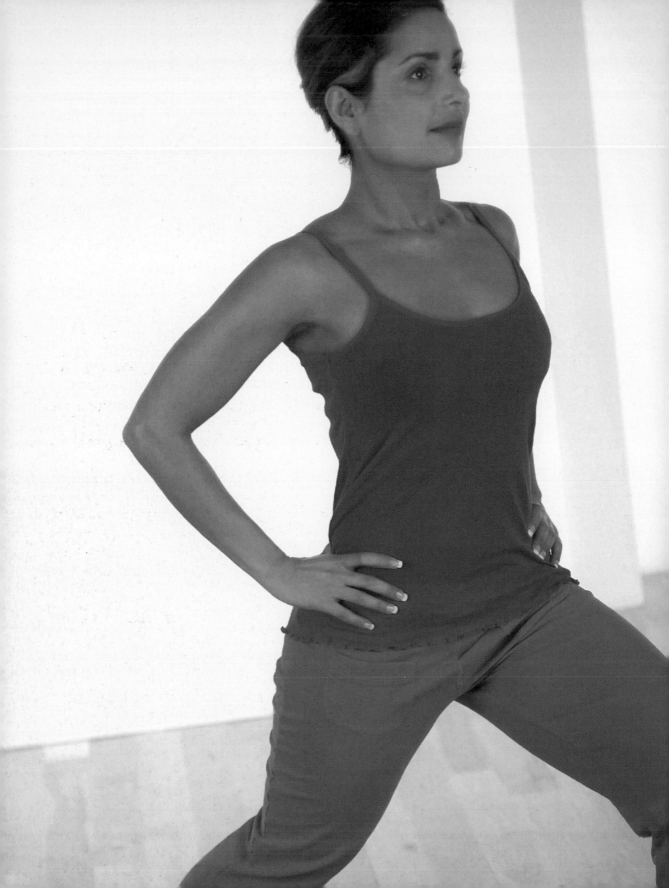

STRETCHES FOR DAILY ACTIVITIES

Considering the demands we place on our overworked bodies, they serve us remarkably well. It is easy to forget how mundane, day-to-day tasks such as working at a computer, driving, and talking on the telephone all take a physical toll on the body. Here I present essential stretches to get you through your day. Whether you garden, sit at a computer, or spend long periods on your feet, there are stretches here for you. A well-chosen stretch can ease muscle aches and pains and keep you feeling energized throughout the day. Think of stretching as a way of rewarding your body for its unfailing good service to you.

GARDENING

Gardening and outdoor work are not as mundane as one might think. Reaching and leaning can mean that the back holds many awkward positions. Pruning works the muscles in the forearms and hands. Kneeling and repeated bending of the knees can irritate the IT bands, the tendons that run from the hips to the shins.

STRETCHING HELPS TO:
• **restore** the natural curve of the lower back and prevent pain caused by leaning over. • **increase circulation** to the knees by improving the flexibility of the hips.

LOWER BACK FIST PRESS

This stretch is essential for gardeners as it realigns the discs in the lower back, which helps to relieve strain on them. Focus the effect by tightening your abdominals and lifting your groin.

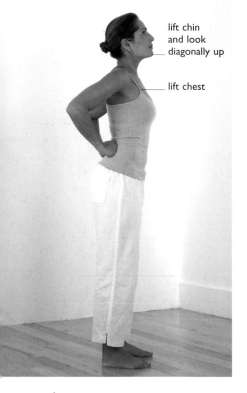

lift chin and look diagonally up

lift chest

1 Stand with your feet hip-width apart. Make two fists with your hands and press them firmly into your lower back as you tighten your abdominals.

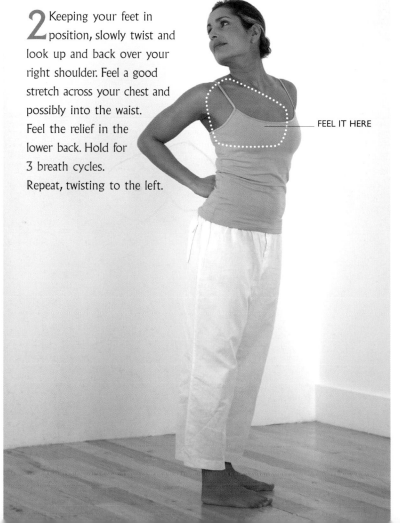

2 Keeping your feet in position, slowly twist and look up and back over your right shoulder. Feel a good stretch across your chest and possibly into the waist. Feel the relief in the lower back. Hold for 3 breath cycles. Repeat, twisting to the left.

FEEL IT HERE

WRIST CIRCLES

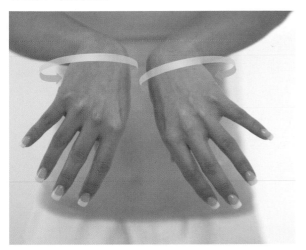

Hold your arms still as you circle both hands at the wrists. Circle 10 times in each direction.

KNEE CIRCLES

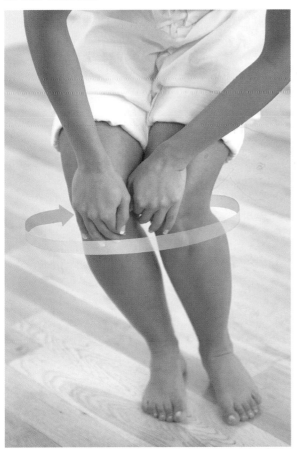

Pull your navel into your spine. Reach down and place one hand on each knee. Allow your knees to support some of your upper body weight. Keep your back as straight as you can by leaning over from the hips. Gently circle your knees. Breathe easily as you circle 6 times in each direction.

MINI CATALOGUE

Perform these stretches to help protect your back and legs. You could also add the hand exercises on page 107.

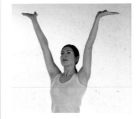

arms open *p29*
hold for 3 breath cycles

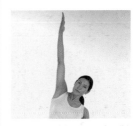

standing side stretch *p31*
hold for 4 breath cycles
repeat on other side

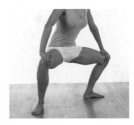

inner thigh squat *p45*
hold for 3 breath cycles

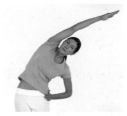

side hip stretch *p43*
hold for 4 breath cycles
repeat on other side

COMPUTER USE

The arteries that supply oxygen to the nerves in our neck and shoulders run through a narrow space between the collar bone and first rib. Tensing up to focus forwards on our work compresses this area, causing tired muscles as well as nerve and tendon irritation. Do at least two of these stretches every half an hour.

STRETCHING HELPS TO:

- **prevent nerve damage** from repetitive mouse and keyboard use.
- **relieve tension build-up** in the shoulders, back, and arms.
- **prevent eye strain** and headaches by refreshing the eyes.

CHAIR TILT

Sit slightly forwards on a chair, your feet firmly planted on the floor. Reach your hands back and hold on to the back of your seat. If you can, lean back and use the chair back to brace you. Look diagonally upwards and open your chest. Hold for 3 breath cycles, then relax.

FEEL IT HERE

lift chest

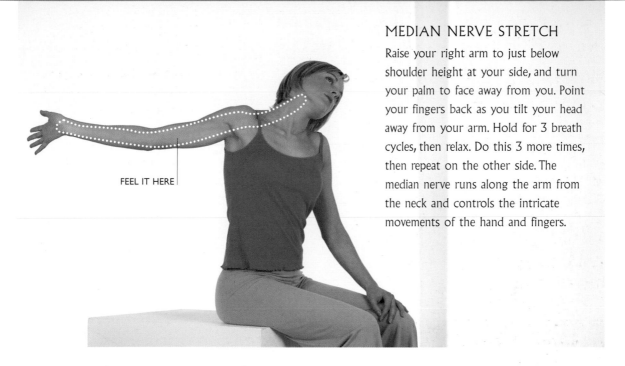

FEEL IT HERE

MEDIAN NERVE STRETCH

Raise your right arm to just below shoulder height at your side, and turn your palm to face away from you. Point your fingers back as you tilt your head away from your arm. Hold for 3 breath cycles, then relax. Do this 3 more times, then repeat on the other side. The median nerve runs along the arm from the neck and controls the intricate movements of the hand and fingers.

ULNAR NERVE STRETCH

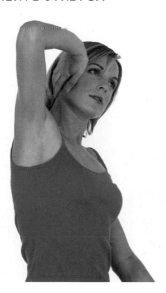

Raise your right hand and rest it against your right cheek with fingers pointing downwards. Tilt your left ear towards your left shoulder. Hold for 3 breath cycles, then relax. Do this 3 more times, then repeat on the other side. This stretch will help to keep your grip strong.

RADIAL NERVE STRETCH

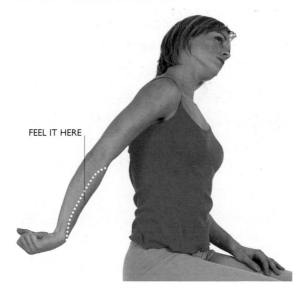

FEEL IT HERE

Make a fist and bend it inwards towards the forearm. Straighten your elbow and lift your hand behind you. Hold for 2 breath cycles, then relax. Do this 3 more times, then repeat on the other hand. Although you feel it in the forearm, it eases the entire radial nerve to the hand.

SEATED COBRA

A great upper back relaxer, this reverses the forwards-slumping posture of rounded shoulders. Be sure to lengthen the back of your neck and reach out through the top of your head rather than just cocking it back in step 2.

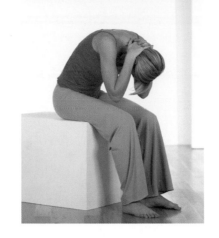

1 Sit towards the back of a chair and plant your feet firmly on the floor. Lean forwards and clasp your hands behind your neck.

pull elbows back

EAR PULL

2 Scoop down and forwards, opening your elbows and reaching the tops of your ears towards the ceiling. Hold for 1 breath cycle, then relax. Repeat this 3 times.

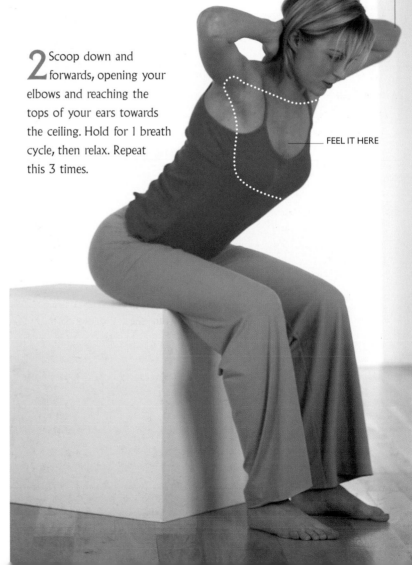

FEEL IT HERE

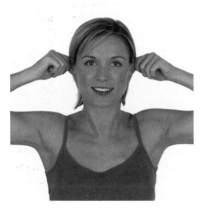

Diffuse tension by pinching the hard cartilage in each of your ears and gently pulling upwards. Hold for 2 breath cycles, then release and repeat again. Try yawning as you breathe to help release tight jaw muscles that can contribute to headache pain.

CLASPED HAND ROTATIONS

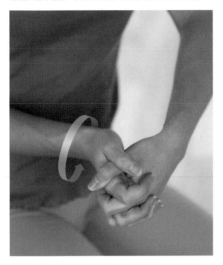

Tuck your right elbow into your body. Interlace your fingers, and use your left hand to help you to make circles with your right wrist. Circle 10 times in each direction. Repeat with the other hand.

FORCEFUL EXHALATION

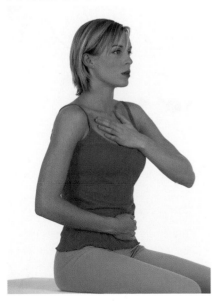

CLASPED HAND CIRCLES

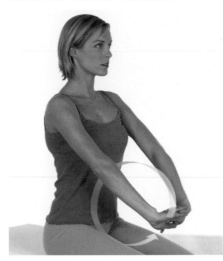

Sit up straight, with head up and feet firmly planted on the floor. Interlace your fingers and make vertical circling motions with your hands, moving up, in towards yourself, down, then forwards 5 times. Then change direction and repeat 5 times. Consciously inhale and exhale throughout.

Sit comfortably with one hand on your chest, the other on your stomach. Slowly but forcefully exhale through your open mouth for a count of 15 seconds. Feel as if you are wringing out a wet cloth with your chest. Breathe normally for 2 breath cycles, then repeat the forceful exhalation once more. This is extremely effective for relieving tense shoulders – it activates the diaphragm so strongly that it causes the upper shoulders and base of the neck to relax.

MINI CATALOGUE

Your eyes and neck need regular stretching when working at a computer for long periods – so do your waist, ribs, and legs.

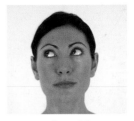

eye stretches *p23*
repeat sequence once

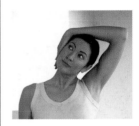

neck stretch *p24*
hold for 2 breath cycles;
repeat on other side

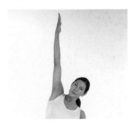

standing side stretch *p31*
hold for 4 breath cycles;
repeat on other side

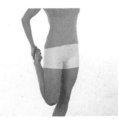

standing quad stretch *p44*
hold for 3 breath cycles;
repeat on other leg

LONG DRIVES

Driving for long periods can be hard on the body. The seats tend to round the lower back out of its natural arch, which strains the muscles. Working the pedals tightens the legs, while gripping the wheel and focusing forwards create tension in the neck, shoulders, and upper back. Try to take a stretching break every 90 minutes.

STRETCHING HELPS TO:

- **preserve back health** – car seats encourage slumped sitting, which can strain muscles and endanger discs.
- **lengthen leg muscles** and help to prevent chronic knee pain.

GLUTEAL STRETCH

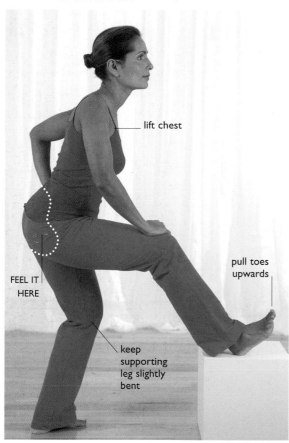

lift chest

pull toes upwards

FEEL IT HERE

keep supporting leg slightly bent

With the car door open, reach your right foot up on to the running board; bend both knees slightly. Lean forwards and hold on to either your leg or the car to brace yourself. Gently push back into the right side of your pelvis. Hold for 3 breath cycles. Repeat with the other leg.

DRIVER'S HAMSTRING STRETCH

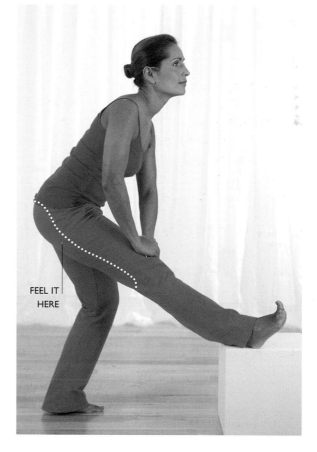

FEEL IT HERE

With the car door open, reach your right foot up on to the running board and pull your toes upwards. Place both hands on your right thigh. Keep your leg as straight as possible as you lean forwards over it. Hold for 3 breath cycles, then repeat with the other leg.

HIP SWAY

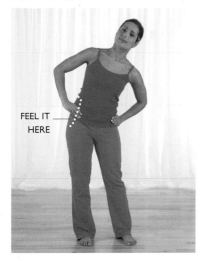

FEEL IT HERE

Stand with feet hip-width apart, your hands on your hips. Gently tuck your pelvis under and use your left hand to push your hips to the right. Take care not to lean back. Hold for 3 breath cycles, then repeat, pushing your hips to the left.

BACKWARDS PRAYER

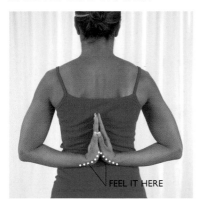

FEEL IT HERE

Stand straight and roll your shoulders up and back. Reach your hands behind you and assume a prayer position in the small of your back. Hold for 3 breath cycles.

STANDING BACK STRETCH

Stand up straight. Place your hands, fingers pointing down, on your lower back. Pull your navel into your spine as you press your hands forwards. Tuck your chin into your chest, but also lift your ribcage upwards. Hold for 3 breath cycles.

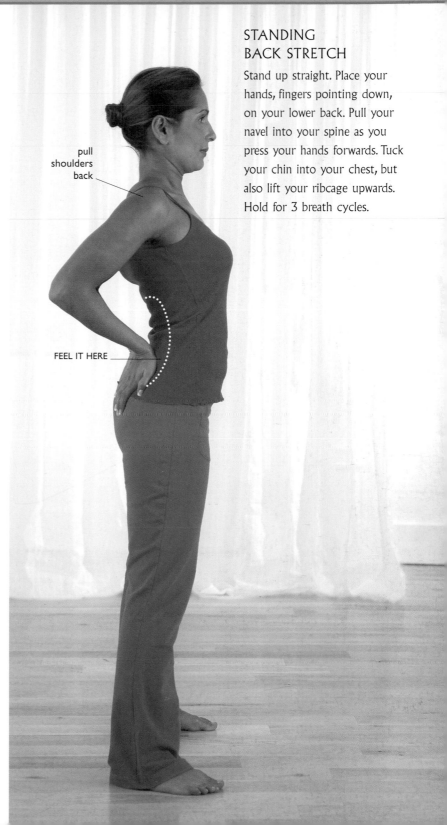

pull shoulders back

FEEL IT HERE

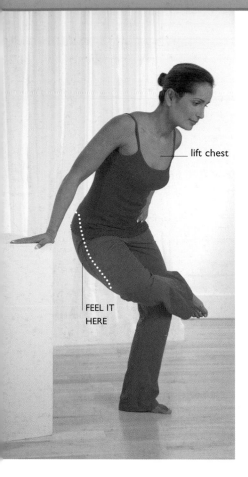

lift chest

FEEL IT
HERE

CALF STRETCH

Place the ball of your right foot
on the running board and let
your heel drop down as you lean
forwards into your foot. Place
both hands on your knee and
press downwards to increase the
stretch. Hold for 3 breath cycles.
Repeat on the other leg.

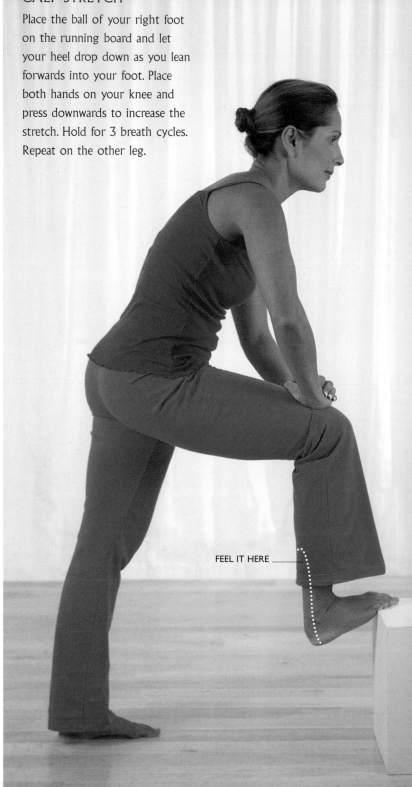

FEEL IT HERE

IT BAND STRETCH

Hold on to the car for balance with
your right hand, and place your left
hand on your hip. Cross your right
foot over your left knee. Pull your
navel in and lean forwards from
your hips, keeping your back flat
to concentrate the stretch in your
right hip and side of thigh. Hold
for 3 breath cycles, then repeat on
the other side.

TWIST PUNCH

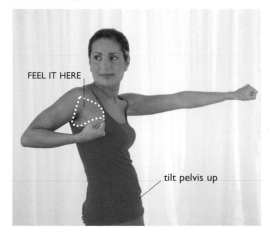

FEEL IT HERE

tilt pelvis up

Stand up tall with feet shoulder-width apart. Make two fists. Punch forwards with your left fist as you pull back with your right elbow and look behind you. Then reverse it, punching your right fist forwards. Repeat each left/right set 6 times. Perform this slowly to stretch under the shoulders and more quickly to invigorate.

HUG WITH HEAD BOW

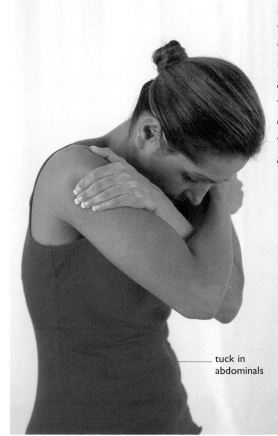

tuck in abdominals

Either stand or sit. Cross your hands and tightly hug your shoulders. Round over, making your chest concave, and bow your head. Pull your chin in towards your chest. Feel the space between your shoulder blades open, and hold for 4 breath cycles.

MINI CATALOGUE

Stuck at the lights or in a sea of traffic? Diffuse tension by performing these simple stretches while in your seat.

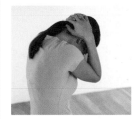

upper back forward stretch *p32*
hold for 2 breath cycles

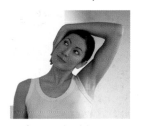

neck stretch *p24*
hold for 2 breath cycles; repeat on other side

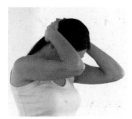

roll-down stretch *p25*
hold for 2 breath cycles

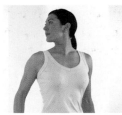

seated head turn *p25*
hold for 2 breath cycles; repeat on other side

FLIGHTS

Flights pose similar problems for the body to long drives – in both cases you are confined to a small seat with limited leg room. Two additional problems on a plane are the physical vibrations, which are associated with back problems, and dehydration, which parches the body's tissues. Perform these stretches every hour, if possible.

STRETCHING HELPS TO:

- **increase circulation**, which may prevent blood clots in the legs from cabin pressure.
- **relieve neck and shoulder** stiffness and pain that may result from sitting in ill-fitting seats.

SEATED REACH-UP

You may have limited leg room, but the space above you is usually available. Take advantage of it by performing this upper body and arm stretch.

2 Now reach your hands above your head. Press your palms upwards as you squeeze your elbows in towards your ears. Hold for 3 breath cycles, then relax.

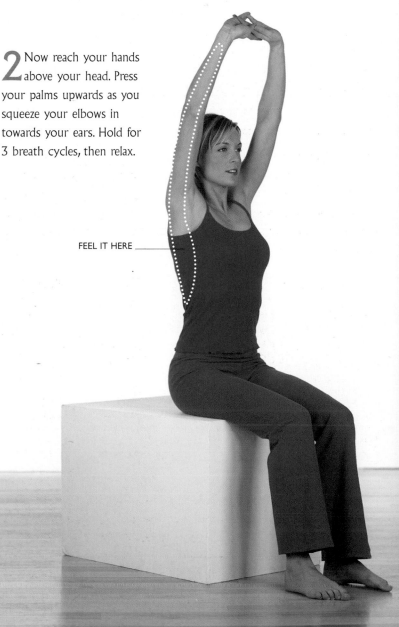

FEEL IT HERE

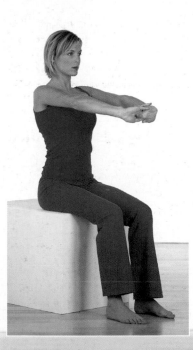

1 Clasp your hands in front of you and turn your palms to face outwards. Stretch your hands forwards. Hold for 3 breath cycles.

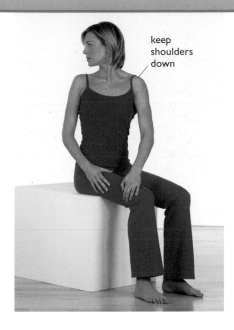

keep shoulders down

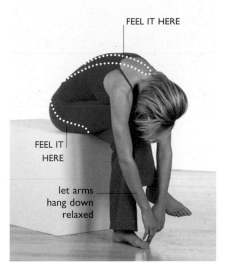

FEEL IT HERE

FEEL IT HERE

let arms hang down relaxed

SEATED BACK TWIST

Sit up straight. Place your left hand on the outside of your right thigh, or the arm rest. "Wind up" your spine, using your abdominal and back muscles. Look around to your right and hold for 2 breath cycles. Release; repeat on the other side.

CROSS-LEGGED HANG

Sit and cross one leg over the other. Lean forwards, letting your head fall towards the floor. Feel the stretch in your back and spine, and hold for 2 breath cycles. Roll up, then repeat with legs crossed the other way.

MINI CATALOGUE

These standing stretches target the legs, waist, and feet. Perform them before boarding the plane, or in the aisle during the flight.

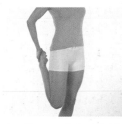

standing quad stretch *p44*
hold for 3 breath cycles; repeat on other leg

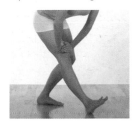

standing hamstring *p46*
hold for 3 breath cycles; repeat on other leg

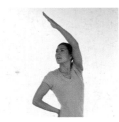

standing waist twist *p40*
hold for 2 breath cycles; repeat on other side

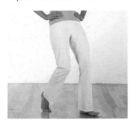

front hip stretch *p42*
hold for 3 breath cycles; repeat on other side

FOOT CIRCLES

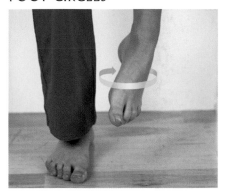

PENDULUM HEAD

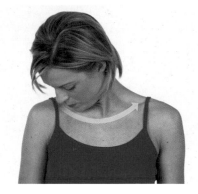

Ensure that you have sufficient room to move your feet. Slowly circle one foot so that you feel the stretch up into your ankles and calves. Circle 10 times in each direction. Repeat with the other foot.

Tuck your chin in towards your chest and point your nose towards the floor. Slowly move your chin from side to side against your chest. Feel the stretch in the back of your neck. Repeat 6 times.

LONG WALKS

Protect your stride and your feet with these stretches. The lunge targets the muscles in the legs and hips, but the soles of the feet and shins need special attention too. An unpleasant yet common complaint, plantar fasciitis, which causes pain in the sole and heel of the foot, can simply be prevented with these stretches.

STRETCHING HELPS TO:

- **prevent leg swelling** and associated feelings of leg heaviness and pain.
- **preserve and improve** a walker's stride length by elongating the leg muscles.

WALKER'S LUNGE

Ensure that your hips face forwards to get the full benefit of this stretch. If your hips twist, you'll get an unbalanced stretch.

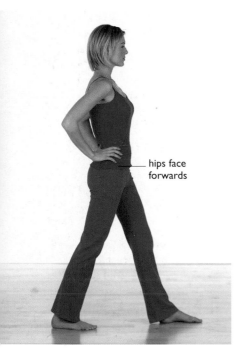

hips face forwards

1 Stand up straight, tighten your abdominals, and lift your chest. With hands on hips, step your left leg forwards. Keep your hips straight and your back heel down.

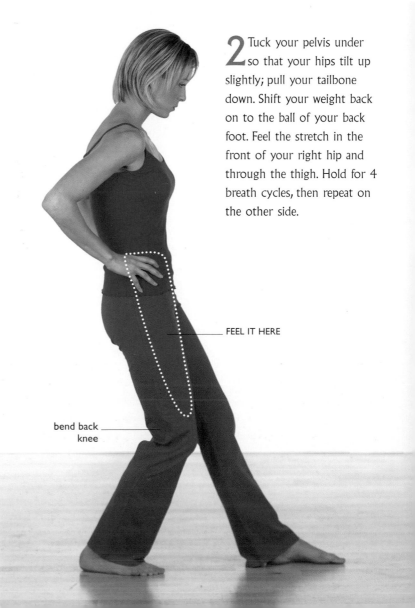

FEEL IT HERE

bend back knee

2 Tuck your pelvis under so that your hips tilt up slightly; pull your tailbone down. Shift your weight back on to the ball of your back foot. Feel the stretch in the front of your right hip and through the thigh. Hold for 4 breath cycles, then repeat on the other side.

BENT-OVER HIP STRETCH

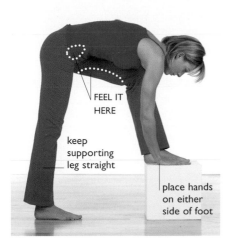

FEEL IT HERE

keep supporting leg straight

place hands on either side of foot

Stand up straight and tighten your abdominals. Bend your leg and prop your foot up on a raised support such as a step. Tuck your pelvis under and lean over your bent leg. Hold for 4 breath cycles. Repeat on the other leg.

FOOT TWIST

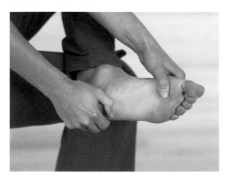

Sit and rest your left foot on your right thigh. Hold the ball of your foot with one hand and the heel with the other. Hold the heel still as you twist the top of the foot one way for 1 breath and the other way for another breath. Repeat, twisting each way 3 times.

BEACH WALK FOOT STRETCH

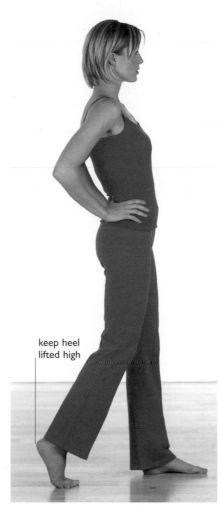

keep heel lifted high

Beach walking can cause pain in the heels and soles of the feet. Perform this stretch barefoot, before and after a walk. Step one foot back behind you and lift the heel upwards so that your toes bend back and your weight is on the ball of your foot. Keeping the heel lifted, press back into your toes until you feel a stretch into the sole of your foot. This should not be painful. Hold for 3 breath cycles, then repeat on the other foot.

MINI CATALOGUE

Walking on hard city pavements can be tiring. These stretches will provide relief for your feet, legs, and back.

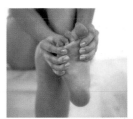

transverse arch p51
repeat both steps 5 times on each foot

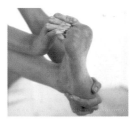

toe bend p51
hold for 3 breath cycles; repeat on other foot

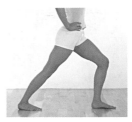

basic lunge p48
hold for 4 breath cycles; repeat on other leg

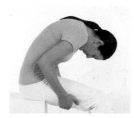

seated head curl p36
hold for 2 breath cycles

LONG TELEPHONE CALLS

Telephone use ranks along with computer use as a cause of muscle tension and nerve irritations. The ulnar nerve, which runs from the hand and up through the elbow, may become tight from bending your arm to hold the phone to your ear. Cradling the phone in the crook of your neck can pinch the nerves there.

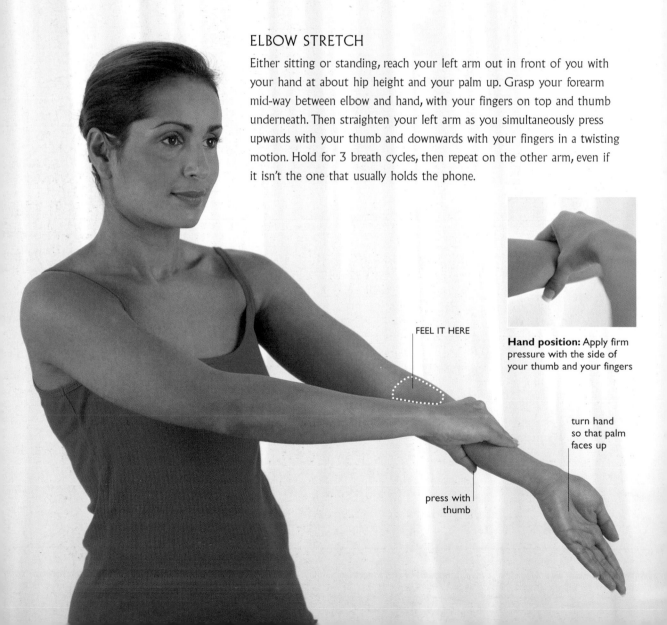

STRETCHING HELPS TO:

- **counteract** the tendency to round the shoulders forwards, which causes pinched nerves and upper back pain.

ELBOW STRETCH

Either sitting or standing, reach your left arm out in front of you with your hand at about hip height and your palm up. Grasp your forearm mid-way between elbow and hand, with your fingers on top and thumb underneath. Then straighten your left arm as you simultaneously press upwards with your thumb and downwards with your fingers in a twisting motion. Hold for 3 breath cycles, then repeat on the other arm, even if it isn't the one that usually holds the phone.

FEEL IT HERE

Hand position: Apply firm pressure with the side of your thumb and your fingers

turn hand so that palm faces up

press with thumb

HANDS-BEHIND-BACK TWIST

We tend to round our shoulders forwards when using the phone. This stretch counteracts that tendency by opening the chest as well as helping to pull the head back so that it aligns over the spine.

MINI CATALOGUE

Long phone conversations wreak havoc on the neck, shoulders, and arms. Some of these stretches can be performed while chatting.

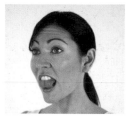

lion stretch *p23*
say "ahhh" for 5 counts

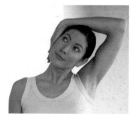

head tilts *p24*
hold for 2 breath cycles each; repeat on other side

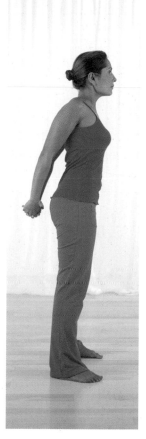

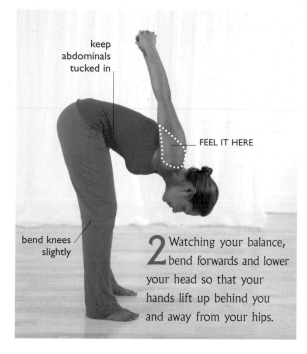

keep abdominals tucked in

FEEL IT HERE

bend knees slightly

2 Watching your balance, bend forwards and lower your head so that your hands lift up behind you and away from your hips.

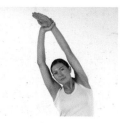

shoulders side *p27*
hold for 4 breath cycles; repeat on other side

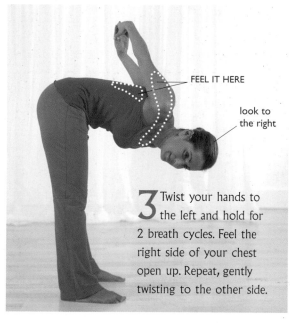

FEEL IT HERE

look to the right

1 Stand straight, with feet hip-width apart. Tighten your abdominals, and pull your navel into your spine. Roll your shoulders up and back, and clasp your hands behind you.

3 Twist your hands to the left and hold for 2 breath cycles. Feel the right side of your chest open up. Repeat, gently twisting to the other side.

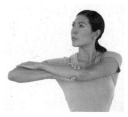

twist, arms crossed *p33*
hold for 2 breath cycles; repeat on other side

STANDING

Queuing, waitressing, shop work, or just wandering around a museum, all take their toll on the muscles in the back, legs, and feet. You can perform these stretches relatively inconspicuously while on your feet, or at home where you can relax. Generally, for the unweighting stretches, lean away from the area of discomfort.

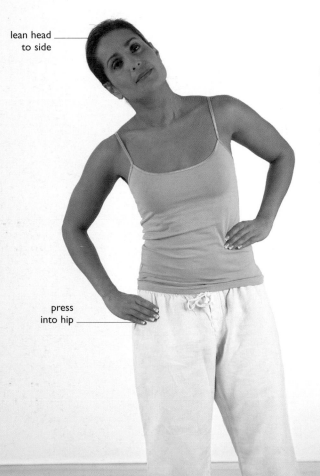

lean head to side

press into hip

LEG UNWEIGHTING

Standing, unweight your left leg by shifting your weight on to your right leg. Place your left hand on your waist and your right hand on your hip. Lift your ribcage up, pull your navel into your spine, and lean your shoulders to the right. Hold for 2 breath cycles, then repeat on the other side, if appropriate. If you suffer from lower back pain on one side, lean away from that side.

ROLLING FEET

This rocking motion is an unweighting technique for the feet. It encourages good posture by helping to re-establish optimum weight distribution over the arches. It doesn't have to be a big motion to have a big effect.

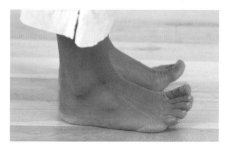 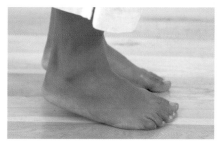

1 Stand up straight and lift your pelvic floor so that it feels as if your spine is being pulled upwards. Gently roll back on your feet, lifting your toes and shifting your weight back on to your heels.

2 Gently roll forwards on your feet, shifting your weight away from your heels and on to your toes. Repeat this rolling motion backwards and forwards about 5 times, or more if desired.

THE THINKER

Prop your right foot up on a support such as a step, stool, doorstop, or curb. Bend your right knee, pull your navel into your spine, and lean forwards. Prop your elbow up on your thigh and rest your chin on your hand. This relieves your right leg while your left leg supports your weight. Repeat with the left foot propped up to relieve pressure on your left leg.

pull stomach in

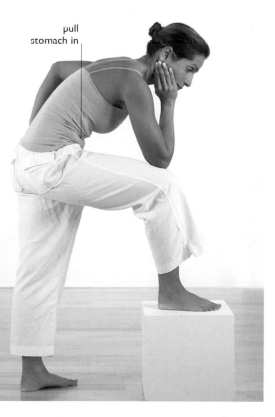

MINI CATALOGUE

Give yourself a lift, and decrease fatigue by adding this sequence of ankle, torso, and foot stretches to your routine.

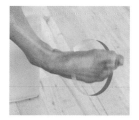

ankle circles *p50*
circle 5 times, each direction; repeat with other foot

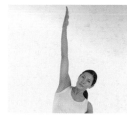

standing side stretch *p31*
hold for 4 breath cycles; repeat on other side

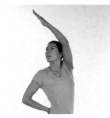

standing waist twist *p40*
hold for 2 breath cycles; repeat on other side

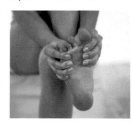

transverse arch *p51*
repeat both steps 5 times on each foot

SITTING

We have a tendency to slump forwards as we get older. Sitting slightly forwards in your chair and gently pulling your buttocks together will help you to elongate your spine and sit up straight. The rule of thumb when sitting for long periods is to stretch regularly, at least every half hour, and before you are uncomfortable.

STRETCHING HELPS TO:
• **decompress** the bottom of the pelvis and lower back, helping to prevent pain and discomfort.   • **restore muscle length** in the hips and thighs, preventing knee pain and problems standing up.

SHOULDER BLADE SQUEEZE

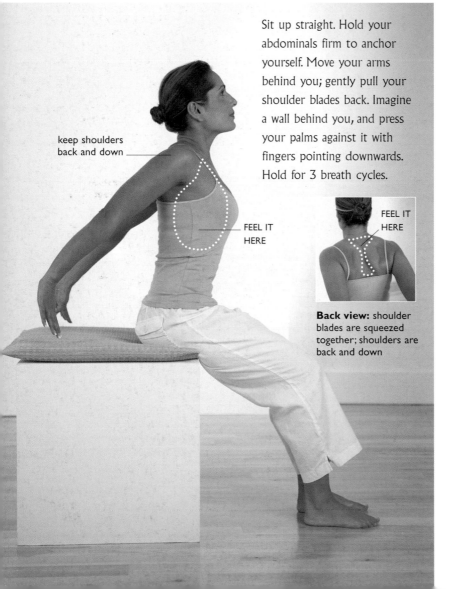

keep shoulders back and down

FEEL IT HERE

Sit up straight. Hold your abdominals firm to anchor yourself. Move your arms behind you; gently pull your shoulder blades back. Imagine a wall behind you, and press your palms against it with fingers pointing downwards. Hold for 3 breath cycles.

FEEL IT HERE

Back view: shoulder blades are squeezed together; shoulders are back and down

HIP TILT

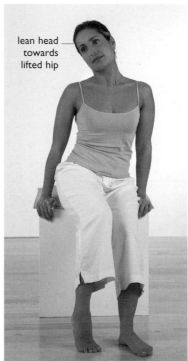

lean head towards lifted hip

Place your hands on either side of you on your seat. Lean to the left, taking the weight off of your right hip bone, and tilt your head to the right. Hold for 1 breath cycle, then repeat, leaning to the right, if appropriate. If you have pain on just one side, only unweight and shift away from that side.

HIP WALK BACK

This stretches the lower back and the muscles in the back of the pelvis, areas that typically become stiff after prolonged periods of sitting.

1 Sit towards the front of your seat. Ensure that you are sitting up straight with your feet flat on the floor. Line up your knees.

2 Press your left hip back into the chair and hold for 1 breath cycle. Then press your right hip back. Perform this 4 times, alternating from side to side and moving backwards.

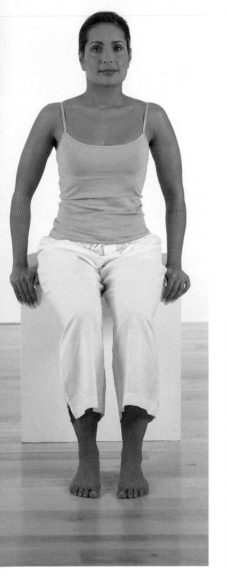

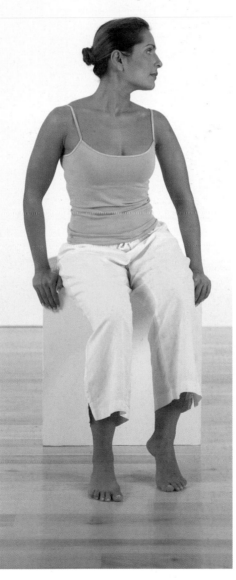

MINI CATALOGUE

These stretches will help to prevent eye and hand strain. They will also give your body a reviving lift if sitting for long periods.

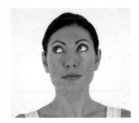

eye stretches *p23*
repeat sequence once

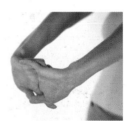

clasped fingers *p28*
hold for 3 breath cycles

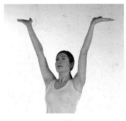

arms open *p29*
hold for 3 breath cycles

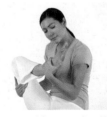

leg-cross hip stretch *p43*
hold for 4 breath cycles;
repeat on other side

LIFTING AND HAULING

First, ensure that your lifting technique is biomechanically sound: keep your back straight, tilt from your hips, and get under the weight so that you can lift with your legs. Whether you are lifting heavy weights, handling a toddler, or moving bags of garden soil, be sure to stretch out muscles that have been put under strain.

STRETCHING HELPS TO:

- **prevent lower back** muscle strain and disc injuries, common complaints after lifting weights.
- **restore normal back** motion after the compressing effect on the spine of lifting a heavy weight.

LUNGE WITH FISTS IN BACK

Step your left foot forwards into a lunge. Press the fists of both hands into your lower back as you lift your chest diagonally upwards. Hold for 3 breath cycles, feeling a good stretch in your calf, lower back, and chest. Repeat with the right foot stepped forwards.

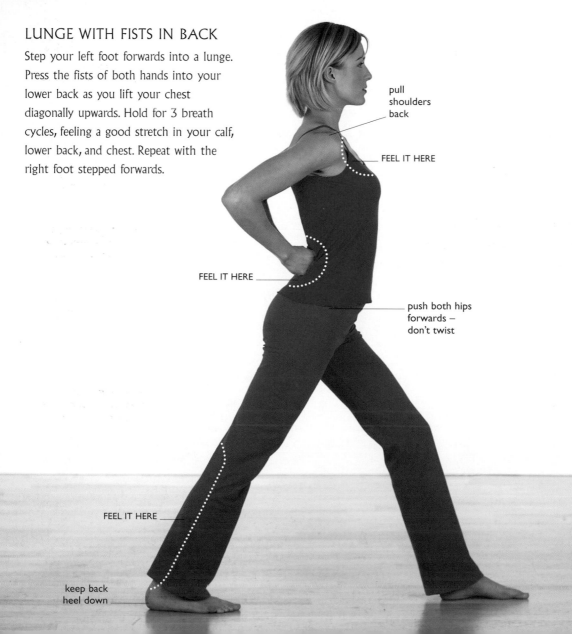

pull shoulders back

FEEL IT HERE

FEEL IT HERE

push both hips forwards – don't twist

FEEL IT HERE

keep back heel down

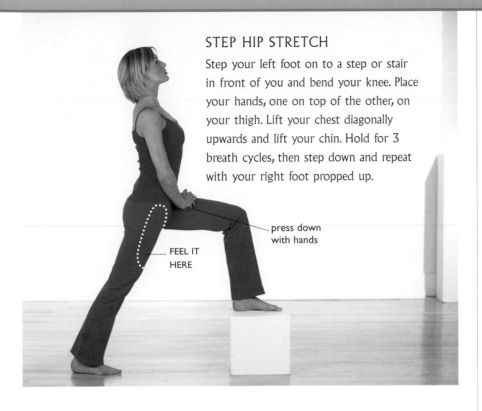

STEP HIP STRETCH

Step your left foot on to a step or stair in front of you and bend your knee. Place your hands, one on top of the other, on your thigh. Lift your chest diagonally upwards and lift your chin. Hold for 3 breath cycles, then step down and repeat with your right foot propped up.

press down with hands

FEEL IT HERE

STANDING BACK TWIST

This twisting stretch benefits the spine and opens the chest, shoulders, and arms. Use your back muscles to twist, and stay as vertical as possible.

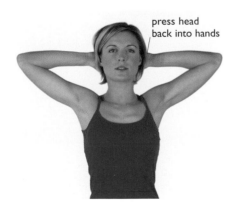

press head back into hands

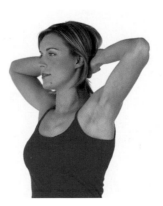

1 Stand with feet shoulder-width apart. Lift your pelvic floor and pull your navel into your spine. Clasp your hands behind your head and open your elbows so they point out to the sides.

2 Twist to the right. Look to the right as you pull your elbows back and press your head back. Hold for 3 breath cycles, then twist back to the front and repeat, twisting to the left.

MINI CATALOGUE

Be sure to stretch your arms and complete these additional stretches to help restore your upright posture after lifting.

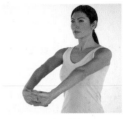

arm stretch *p28*
hold for 3 breath cycles

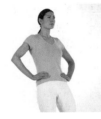

front hip stretch *p42*
hold for 3 breath cycles; repeat on other side

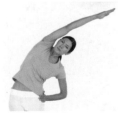

side hip stretch *p43*
hold for 4 breath cycles; repeat on other side

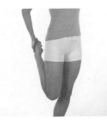

standing quad stretch *p44*
hold for 3 breath cycles; repeat on other leg

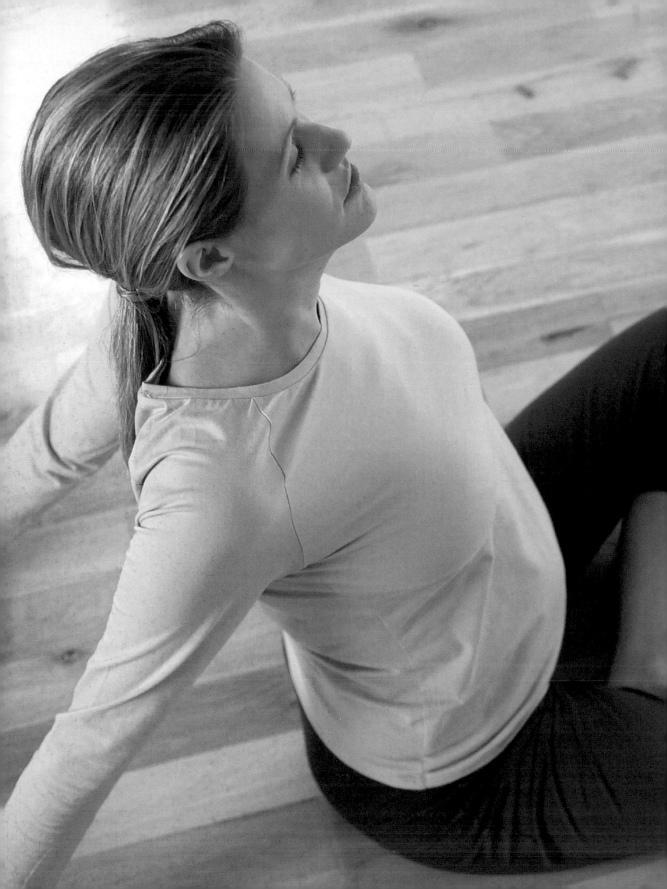

STRETCHES FOR DIFFERENT TIMES OF LIFE

The exercises in this section are designed for those times of life when a gentler approach to stretching is required. During pregnancy, stretching can help maintain flexibility and prepare the body for delivery, but it is important to work within comfortable limits. After pregnancy, gentle stretching can help rebalance your muscles. In later life, the goal is to keep the whole body supple, but particularly the spine and hands. Respect your body's limitations, but rely on regular stretching to keep you active and energized.

PREGNANCY

Muscle tightness in the chest, lower back, and hips is common during pregnancy. As you grow in size, your centre of gravity changes, which can unbalance your posture. Perform these stretches every day to help your flexibility for delivery. For side-lying stretches, place a pillow under your waist to support your back.

CAUTIONS AND TIPS

- **Confirm** with your doctor that it is safe for you to perform these stretches.
- **Listen to your body** and don't overdo it. Stretch only as far as is comfortable.

WIDE SQUAT

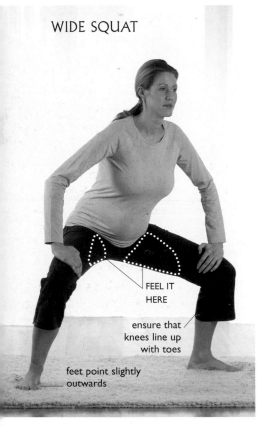

FEEL IT HERE

ensure that knees line up with toes

feet point slightly outwards

Step your feet a comfortable distance apart. Keeping your hips tucked under, and supporting yourself by placing your hands on your thighs, slowly squat down. Feel a gentle stretch in your inner thighs. Hold for 4 breath cycles. Work up to repeating this 3 times.

GENTLE GLUTE STRETCH

Sit on the floor. Extend your right leg out to the side and bend your left knee, bringing your foot towards the groin. Place your right hand in your lower back and reach your left hand towards your right leg, touching it if you can. There should be no pain in your lower back or bent knee. Hold for 3 breath cycles, then repeat on the other side.

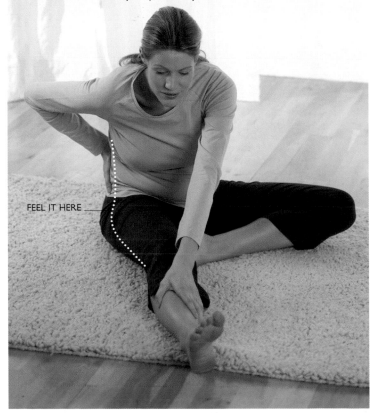

FEEL IT HERE

CROSS-LEGGED CHEST LIFT

Sit comfortably on the floor and cross your legs. Reach back with both your hands and support yourself on your fingertips, keeping your fingers slightly bent. Exhale and press down gently on your hands as you lift up your chest. Look up diagonally and breath for 4 breath cycles, then relax down. Repeat 2 more times.

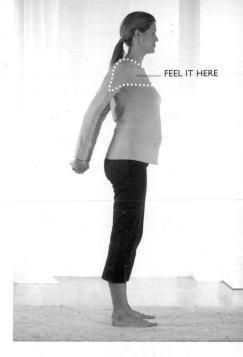

FEEL IT HERE

CLASPED HANDS BACK

Hold your hips steady by tightening your buttocks. Clasp your hands behind you. Roll your shoulders back and pull your hands down towards your feet. Feel a stretch across your chest and into your shoulders. Hold for 4 breath cycles, then relax out of the position.

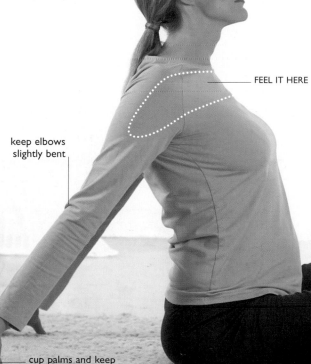

FEEL IT HERE

keep elbows slightly bent

cup palms and keep fingers slightly bent

LYING HAMSTRING STRETCH

Lie on your left side with a pillow under your waist. Slightly bend your left leg. Straighten your right leg in front of you, grasp it at the top of the calf, and pull it towards your chest. Feel a stretch along the back of your leg and hold for 4 breath cycles. Repeat on the other side.

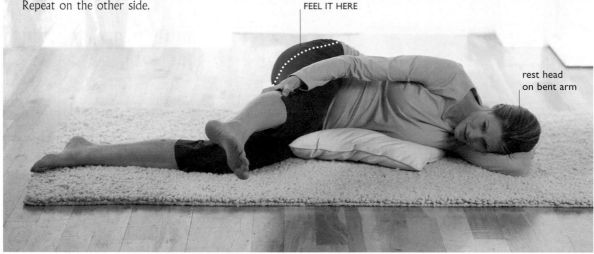

FEEL IT HERE

rest head on bent arm

LYING INNER THIGH STRETCH

Lie on your left side with a pillow under your waist. Slightly bend both legs. Straighten your right leg, grasp it inside the thigh, and open it, pushing your right hip forwards. Feel a stretch along the inside of your thighs, and hold for 3 breath cycles. Repeat on the other side.

FEEL IT HERE

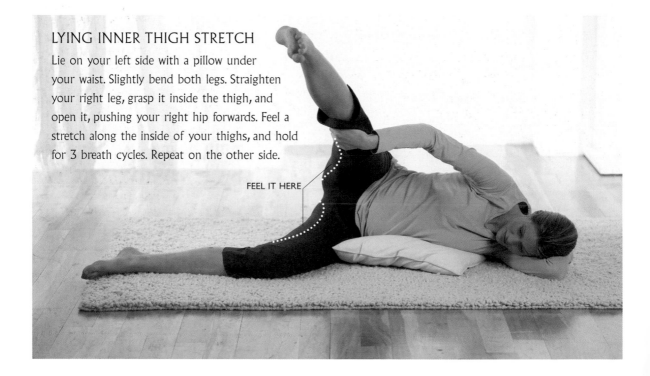

LYING QUAD STRETCH

Lie on your left side with a pillow under your waist. Slightly bend your left leg. Tuck your pelvis under as you reach back to grasp your right ankle or shin and gently pull. Feel a comfortable stretch in the front of your right thigh; hold for 3 breath cycles. Repeat on the other side.

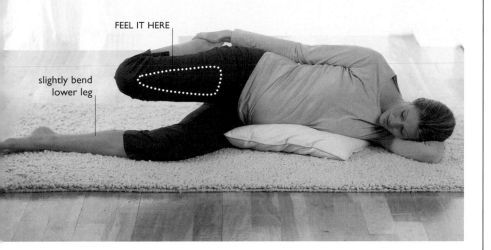

FEEL IT HERE

slightly bend lower leg

CROSSOVER LEG TWIST STRETCH

Lie comfortably on your back. Press your lower back into the floor, bend your right leg, and cross it over your left. Reach your arms out to the sides, and relax into the stretch. Hold for 4 breath cycles, then repeat with your left leg crossed over your right.

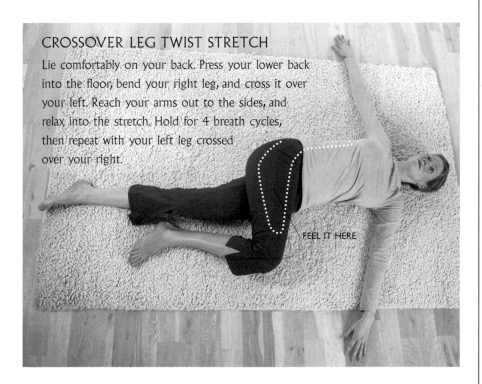

FEEL IT HERE

MINI CATALOGUE

Stretch your jaws, which tighten with your changing centre of gravity. Keep opening your chest, upper ribs, and calves too.

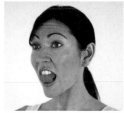

lion stretch *p23*
say "ahhh" for 5 counts

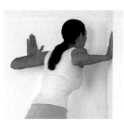

corner chest stretch *p30*
hold for 4 breath cycles

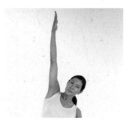

standing side stretch *p31*
hold for 4 breath cycles;
repeat on other side

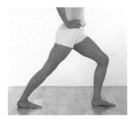

basic lunge *p48*
hold for 4 breath cycles;
repeat on other leg

POST-PREGNANCY

Practise these simple stretches every day to help open the muscles in the lower back and chest, which may have tightened during pregnancy. Your centre of gravity is shifting back to its pre-pregnancy posture; these stretches will help you to regain normal movement as well as re-train and re-balance your body.

GENTLE HAMSTRING

Protect your lower back by tightening your abdominals as you pull your thigh to your chest.

1 Lie on your back and place both feet on the floor, knees slightly bent. Exhale, press your lower back into the floor, and gently pull your left knee towards your chest.

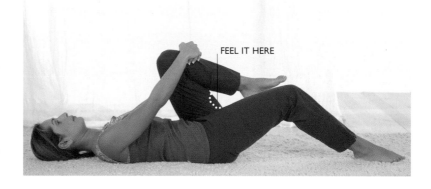

FEEL IT HERE

2 First straighten your right leg, then your left. Hold your left thigh and calf and pull your leg very gently towards you. Hold for 4 breath cycles, feeling a good stretch down the back of your left leg. Then carefully lower your leg and repeat steps 1–2 on the other side.

FEEL IT HERE

FEEL IT HERE

INTENSIFY THE STRETCH
Flex your left foot; pull your calf towards you with your left hand as you press your thigh with your right hand. Feel the stretch up into the sole of your foot.

press calf down

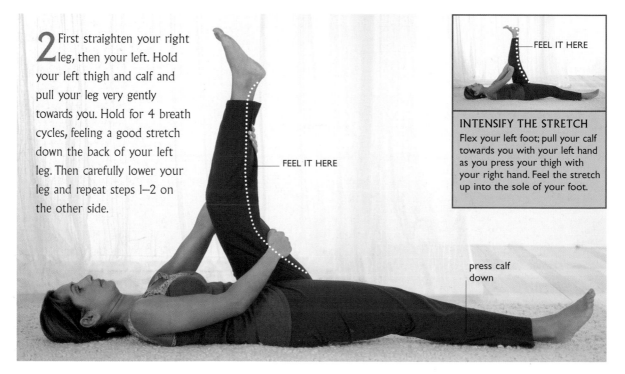

CAT

Start on your hands and knees with your back flat. Inhale as you gently round your back like a scared cat and look at your navel. Imagine a hand lifting your abdomen up towards your spine. Exhale and slowly flatten your back again. Repeat this slow rounding and flattening of your back 5 times.

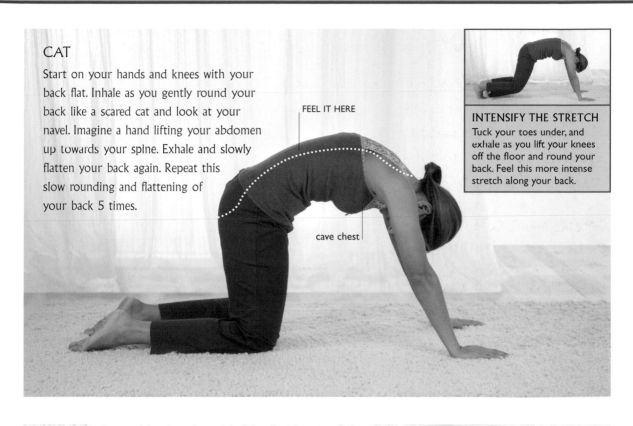

FEEL IT HERE

cave chest

INTENSIFY THE STRETCH
Tuck your toes under, and exhale as you lift your knees off the floor and round your back. Feel this more intense stretch along your back.

CAMEL

Start on your hands and knees with your back flat. Inhale as you lengthen your back, then arch it by tilting your pelvis down. Stretch your head up and back as if trying to get it to touch your bottom. Exhale and slowly flatten your back again. Repeat this slow arching and flattening of your back 5 times.

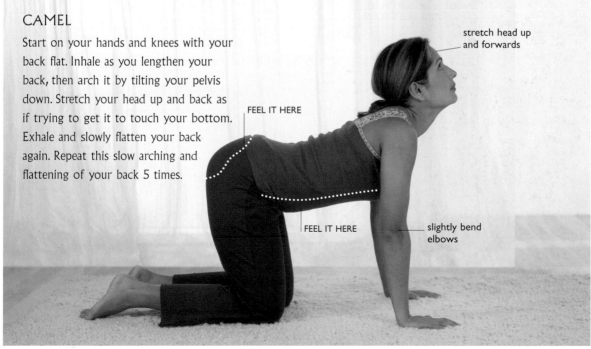

stretch head up and forwards

FEEL IT HERE

FEEL IT HERE

slightly bend elbows

ALLIGATOR

Start on your hands and knees with your back flat. Inhale as you turn your head to the right and look towards your right hip. Feel the stretch along your left side as you slowly exhale. Then inhale and turn your head towards your left hip, exhaling as you stretch your right side. Repeat this moving stretch, right and left, 5 times.

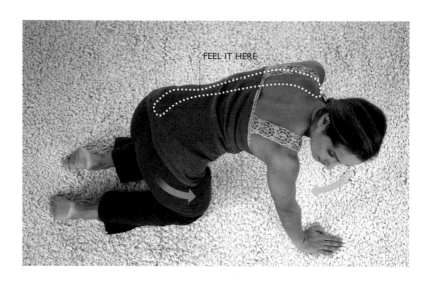

FEEL IT HERE

CONTROLLED TWIST

Keep your head lifted as you twist – imagine that it is suspended by a string from the ceiling.

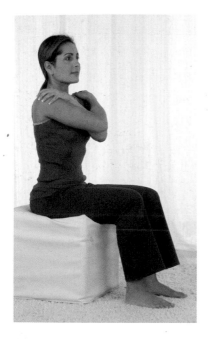

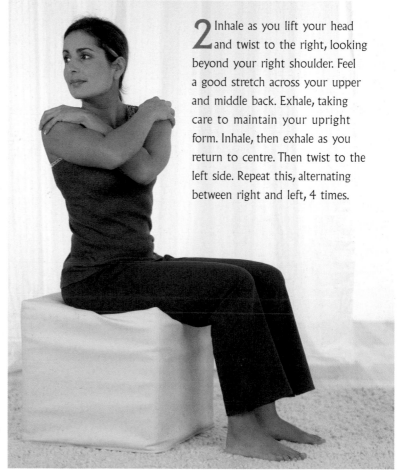

2 Inhale as you lift your head and twist to the right, looking beyond your right shoulder. Feel a good stretch across your upper and middle back. Exhale, taking care to maintain your upright form. Inhale, then exhale as you return to centre. Then twist to the left side. Repeat this, alternating between right and left, 4 times.

1 Sit up straight, with your feet flat on the floor. Place your hands on opposite shoulders.

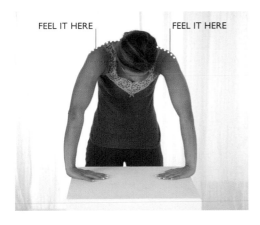

FEEL IT HERE   FEEL IT HERE

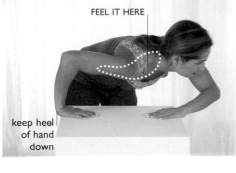

FEEL IT HERE

keep heel of hand down

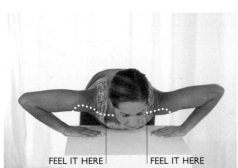

FEEL IT HERE   FEEL IT HERE

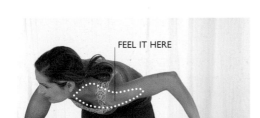

FEEL IT HERE

SHOULDER OVAL STRETCH

Here, moving in an oval shape, you stretch the upper back, armpits, arms, throat, and chest.

1 Place your hands on a surface in front of you. Position them under your shoulders with fingers slightly splayed, pointing inwards. Round your upper back.

2 Hold your abdominals firm, and press your right shoulder towards your left hand. Look to the left, feeling a good stretch in your right shoulder and into your neck.

3 Sweep your breastbone down and around to the centre. Feel the stretch in the fronts of your shoulders and across your chest.

4 Continue making the oval shape as you sweep across to the right, pressing your left shoulder towards your right hand. Look to the right, feeling the stretch in your left shoulder and neck. Repeat steps 1–4, circling in the opposite direction.

MINI CATALOGUE

New mothers need plenty of upper body relief from holding and nursing infants. Be sure to stretch your face, neck, and arms.

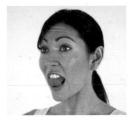

lion stretch *p23*
say "ahhh" for 5 counts

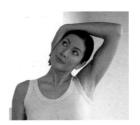

neck stretch *p24*
hold for 2 breath cycles; repeat on other side

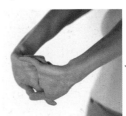

clasped fingers *p28*
hold for 3 breath cycles

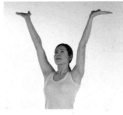

arms open *p29*
hold for 3 breath cycles

LATER IN LIFE

Regular stretching can help to keep us flexible and active well into old age. As we get older, stretching can help to preserve spinal mobility and maintain hand dexterity. If you have trouble with balance, it is possible to perform all of these stretches seated. It's amazing how much can be accomplished in a chair.

SEATED SPINAL ROLL

To help you to round your back as you roll down, pull your navel into your spine and imagine stretching your upper body up and over a fence. As you roll back up, imagine a pull from the seat of your chair.

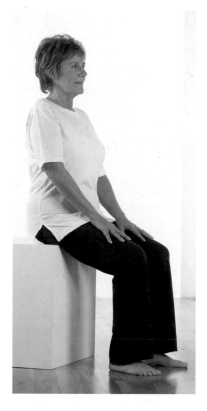

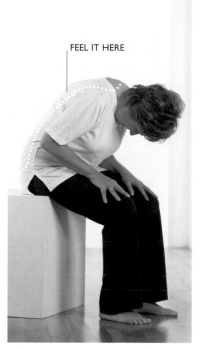

FEEL IT HERE

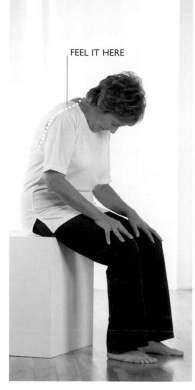

FEEL IT HERE

1 Sit slightly forwards on a chair, your feet flat on the floor, and place your hands on your thighs. Sit up straight and try to align your head over your pelvis.

2 Tuck your chin into your chest and roll down your spine, lowering your head towards your knees. Inhale and pull your navel into your spine as you lower.

3 Exhale, and very slowly roll back up until you are sitting upright again. Repeat steps 1–3 4 times, moving slowly and only going as low as is comfortable.

GENTLE SEATED TWIST

Take care to keep your chest lifted as you perform this stretch. As you twist to the right, sit a bit more heavily on your left hip to prevent you from lifting it off the chair, and vice versa.

1 Sit slightly forwards on a chair, your feet flat on the floor. Sit up straight and place your right hand on your lower back with fingers pointing downwards, and your left hand on your right thigh.

2 Gently turn to the right, and look beyond your right shoulder. Use your left hand to help you to hold the twist. Stay in position for 2 breath cycles, then relax. Switch hand positions and repeat, twisting to the left. Perform once more on each side.

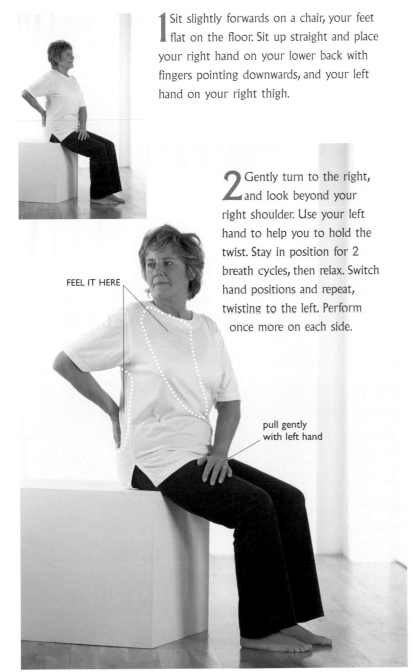

FEEL IT HERE

pull gently with left hand

ANKLE REACH

To help your balance as you lean forwards, open your eyes and consciously focus on your leg.

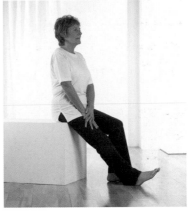

1 Sit slightly forwards on a chair, your back straight. Reach your right heel in front of you, keeping your knee slightly bent. Place both hands on your right thigh.

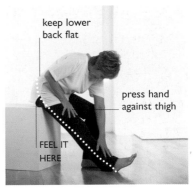

keep lower back flat

press hand against thigh

FEEL IT HERE

2 Lean forwards, keeping your mid-section firm. Twist slightly, reaching your left hand to your right ankle. Hold for 2 breath cycles, then slowly sit up. Repeat on the other side, reaching to your left ankle. Perform once more on each side.

CHEST THRUST

It is possible to perform this stretch seated: begin by sitting slightly forwards on a chair with feet flat on the floor.

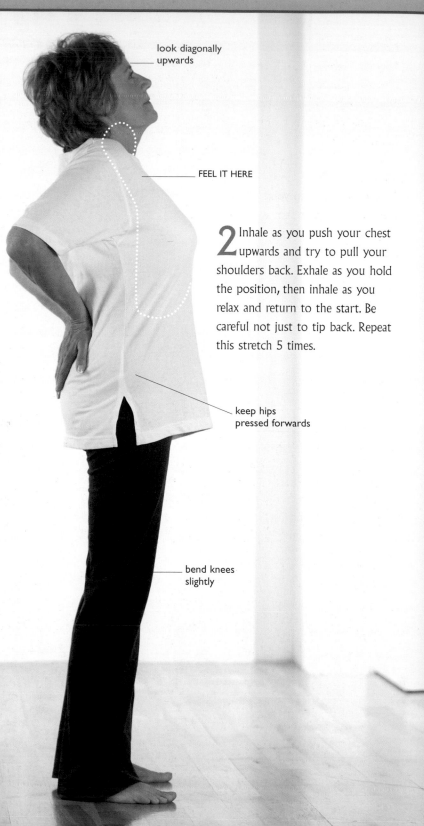

look diagonally upwards

FEEL IT HERE

2 Inhale as you push your chest upwards and try to pull your shoulders back. Exhale as you hold the position, then inhale as you relax and return to the start. Be careful not just to tip back. Repeat this stretch 5 times.

keep hips pressed forwards

bend knees slightly

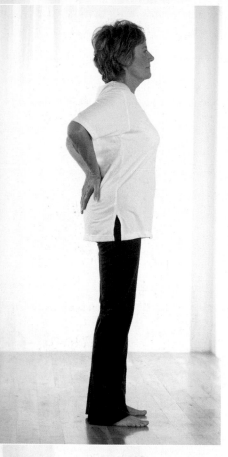

1 Stand with feet hip-width apart and roll your shoulders back to open your chest. Place your hands, fingers pointing downwards, on your lower back.

FINGER SPLAY

Regular stretching can help to keep your hands and fingers flexible. Really open your fingers as wide as you can in step 2.

1 Stretch your arms out in front of you, open your chest, and pull your shoulders back. Flex your wrists and press your palms forwards with fingers together.

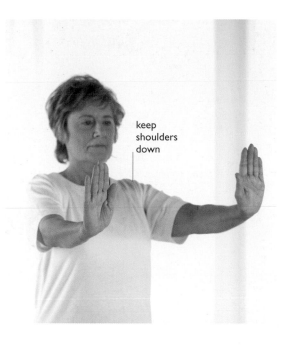

keep shoulders down

2 Open and splay your fingers, spreading them as wide as possible. Then bring your fingers together again. Work up to repeating this stretch, opening and closing your fingers, up to 20 times, if you can.

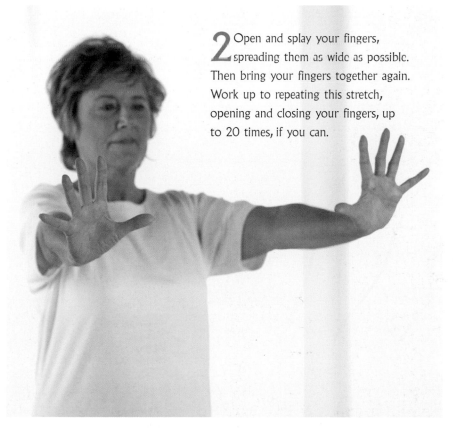

MINI CATALOGUE

Stretching your face, arms, and waist on a regular basis helps to keep you feeling uplifted, energized, and alert.

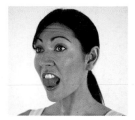

lion stretch *p23*
say "ahhh" for 5 counts

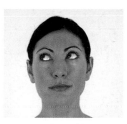

eye stretches *p23*
repeat sequence once

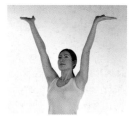

arms open *p29*
hold for 3 breath cycles

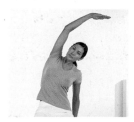

seated waist stretch *p41*
hold for 2 breath cycles;
repeat on other side

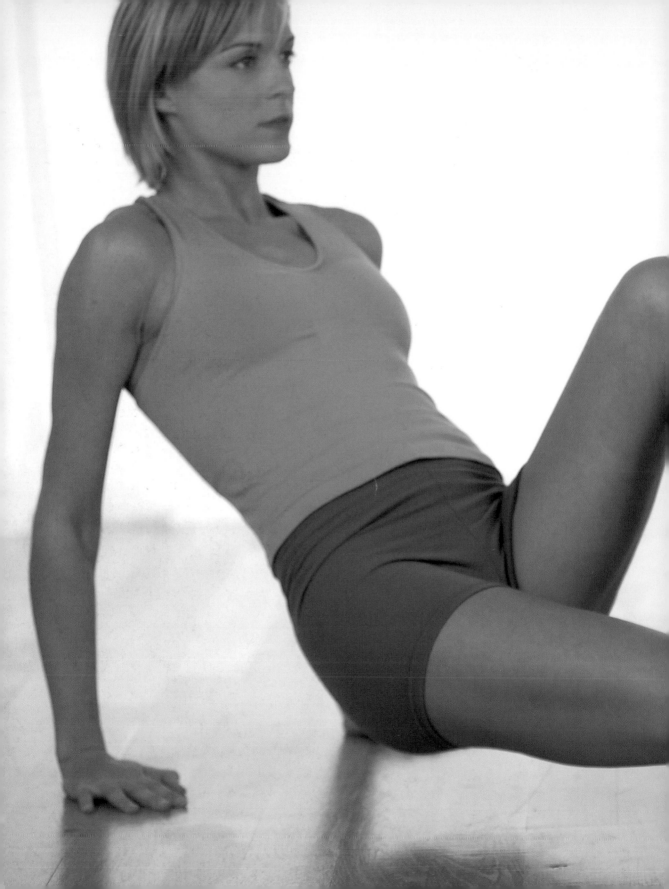

THERAPEUTIC STRETCHES

For those days when you wake up with a crick in your neck, have tired hands from typing, or feel the nagging discomfort of lower back pain, gentle stretching can bring great relief. In this section I present therapeutic stretches for each of the body's typical problem areas. As always, it's important to respect your limits — the goal is not to increase discomfort but to alleviate it. Think of these stretches as preventative measures. What you remedy in the hips and calves can have lasting therapeutic repercussions in the back — everything is interconnected!

NECK AND SHOULDERS

The neck, shoulders, and arms work together as a functional unit. Usually all three areas are involved when there's a problem with any part of the group. As always, exercise caution when stretching anything that is sore, and breathe into the movements. The Towel Rock, below, will work wonders for a crick in the neck.

TOWEL ROCK

If one side of your neck is stiff or achy, begin by rocking away from that side. However, moving in both directions can help to restore range of motion.

1 Start by folding a towel lengthwise into thirds. Lie down with knees bent and place the folded towel behind your head. Hold the longer end on your chest, the other by the side of your face. Press your lower back into the floor.

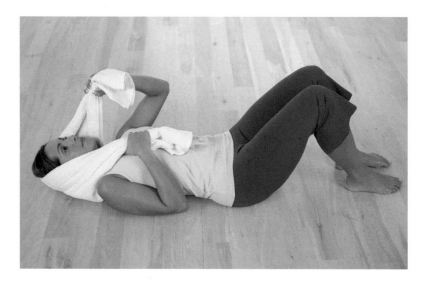

2 Grasp the towel firmly at your chest with your right hand. Gently rock your head to the right by pulling the towel with your left hand. Perform about 10 small and smooth rocking motions. Repeat on the other side, if it is comfortable to do so.

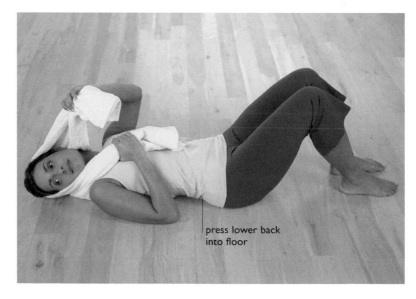

press lower back into floor

ARM CROSS

Be sure to keep your shoulder from riding up towards your ear as you lift your elbow slightly. Ensure that your elbow remains at chest level.

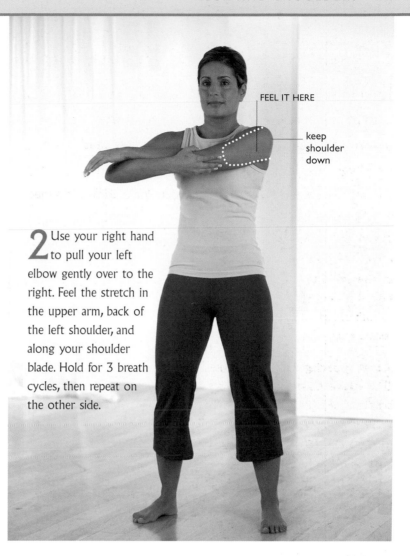

FEEL IT HERE

keep shoulder down

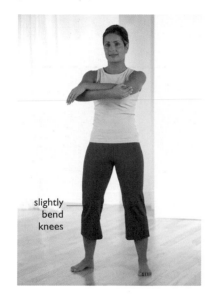

slightly bend knees

1 Stand with feet about shoulder-width apart. Hold your hips steady by pulling your navel into your spine and tightening your buttocks. Cup your left elbow in your right hand, holding under the arm.

2 Use your right hand to pull your left elbow gently over to the right. Feel the stretch in the upper arm, back of the left shoulder, and along your shoulder blade. Hold for 3 breath cycles, then repeat on the other side.

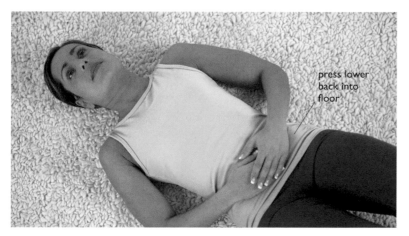

press lower back into floor

FACE CLOCK

Lie on your back with knees bent. Imagine that your face is a clock: 12 is the crown of your head, 3 is your right ear, 6 is your chin, and 9 is your left ear. Roll your head back slightly to 12, then, pressing your head into the floor at each number, slowly move round to 3, 6, 9, and finally 12 again. Perform 4 clock circles in each direction. Breathe normally throughout.

SHOULDER HOLD

This stretch is demonstrated on the right side of the neck, but perform it to the affected side.

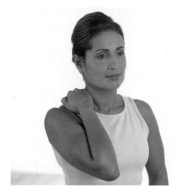

1 Cup your right hand on your trapezius, the meaty area at the top of your shoulder. Gently squeeze with the heel of your hand and pads of your fingers as you pull up.

2 Gently lean your head to the right, resting it on your hand, if you can. Take care not to strain; try to let your head relax. Hold for 6 breath cycles, then slowly raise your head and release your hand. Rub your right shoulder for more relief.

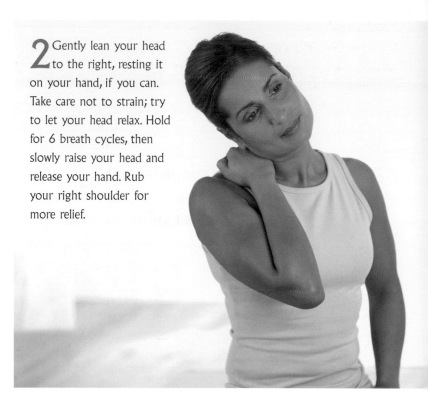

TWO-HANDED HOLD

Try this stretch to relieve the discomfort of a stiff or sore neck.

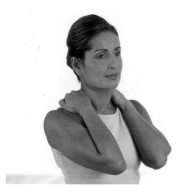

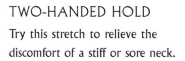

1 Cup both trapezius muscles, the meaty areas at the tops of your shoulders, in your hands. Squeeze with the heels of your hands and pads of your fingers as you pull up.

2 Gently tilt your chin and head downwards, resting your chin on, or close to, your chest. Take care not to strain; try to allow your head to relax. Hold for 6 breath cycles, then slowly raise your head again. Rub both shoulders for more relief.

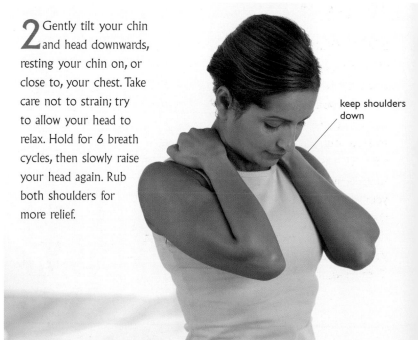

keep shoulders down

PENDULUMS

Use a countertop or table for support when performing this moving shoulder stretch.

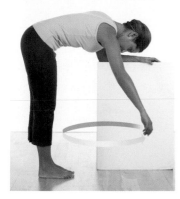

1 Lean forwards, brace yourself on a support, and flatten your back. Allow your right arm to dangle freely, then make 10 circles in each direction. Repeat on the other arm.

2 Relax your right arm and allow it to dangle freely. Gently swing it back and forth like a pendulum. Do this 10 times, then repeat on the other arm.

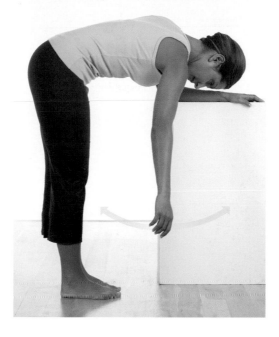

SHOULDER ROLLS

Stand straight and hold your pelvis steady by pulling your navel into your spine and tightening your buttocks. Try to keep your head aligned over your spine as you perform slow shoulder rolls: forwards, up past your ears, then back, squeezing the shoulder blades together. Complete the roll by pulling your shoulders down. Perform 10 shoulder rolls in this manner.

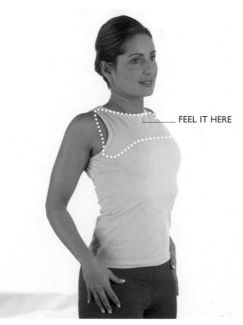

FEEL IT HERE

MINI CATALOGUE

You will be amazed by how much neck and shoulder relief these scalp, face, eye, and hand stretches can provide.

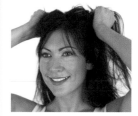

hair pull p22
perform 2 times, moving around the head

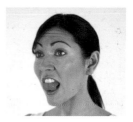

lion stretch p23
say "ahhh" for 5 counts

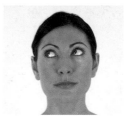

eye stretches p23
repeat sequence once

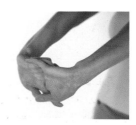

clasped fingers p28
hold for 3 breath cycles

ARMS AND HANDS

You may be surprised to see stretches for the chest and ribcage here, but these are key to resolving repetitive stress injuries (RSI) in the arms and hands. Combined with stretches that aim to correct bad postural habits, they can help to ease compressed nerves and increase circulation to tight muscles and connective tissue.

BALLOONING

This stretches the muscles in the chest and ribcage – consider it to be stretching from the inside out. Keep your back firmly on the floor.

1 Lie on your back with your knees bent. Place one hand on your lower ribcage, thumb between the breasts, and one on your abdomen, thumb at your navel. Breathe in through your nose as you expand your chest and simultaneously tighten your abdominals.

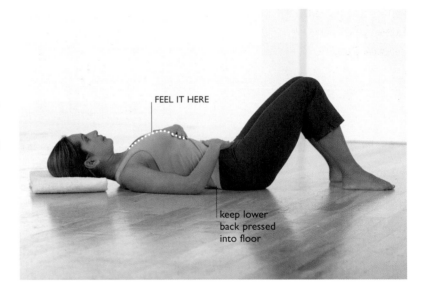

FEEL IT HERE

keep lower back pressed into floor

2 Breathe out through your mouth as you press down on your breastbone and chest, as if squeezing your chest, while you simultaneously expand your abdomen. Take regular breaths in through your nose, then out through your mouth. Repeat 10 times, and work up to 20 repetitions. Be sure not to "buck" the spine back and forth.

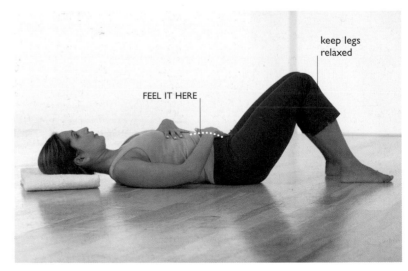

keep legs relaxed

FEEL IT HERE

ARC SWEEP

This opens the muscles in the armpits and the sides of the ribs – stretching these areas can help to prevent RSI problems.

1 Lie on your right side with a pillow or two under your upper body to raise it off the floor a little. Scissor your legs so that the top, left one is back. Extend your arms in front of you with hands together.

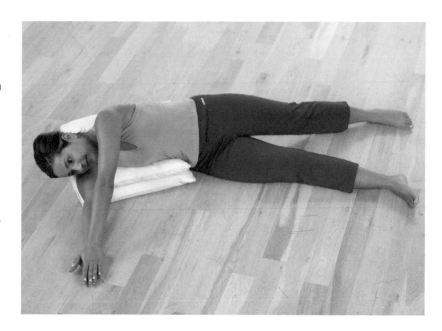

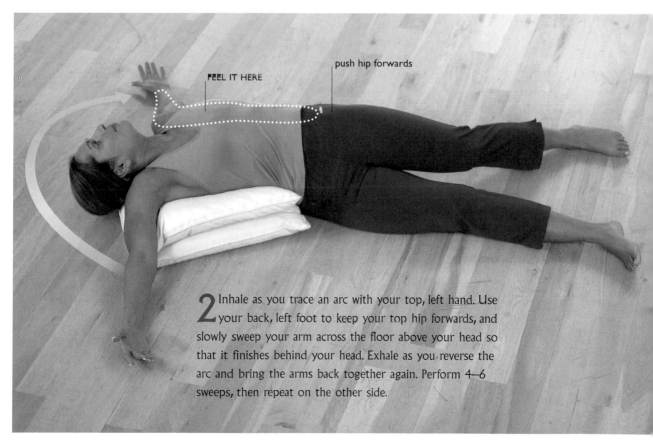

FEEL IT HERE

push hip forwards

2 Inhale as you trace an arc with your top, left hand. Use your back, left foot to keep your top hip forwards, and slowly sweep your arm across the floor above your head so that it finishes behind your head. Exhale as you reverse the arc and bring the arms back together again. Perform 4–6 sweeps, then repeat on the other side.

HAND ROLL

This stretch helps to preserve shoulder flexibility, which deteriorates over time and can be lost when performing repetitive activities with your arms directly in front. The key is to keep your hands curled throughout the stretch.

3 Continue rolling your hands and arms until your elbows point upwards. Then exhale as you unwind your arms. Start from the shoulders, then slowly lower your elbows, straighten your arms, and uncurl your hands and fingers. Repeat this winding and unwinding 3 times.

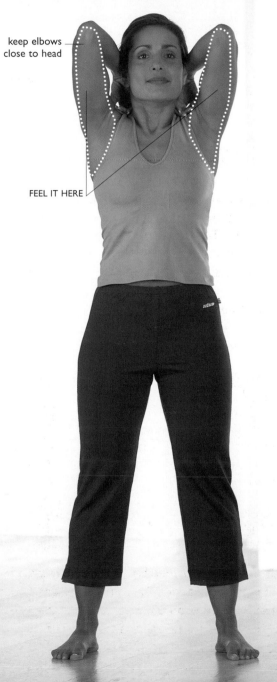

keep elbows close to head

FEEL IT HERE

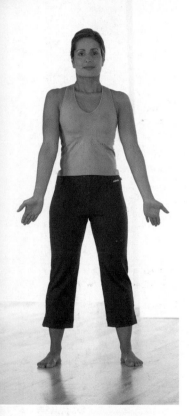

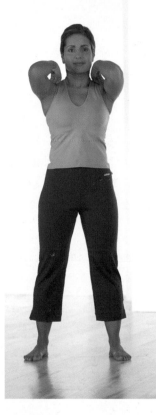

1 Stand up straight, with your feet shoulder-width apart. Hold your hips steady by pulling your navel into your spine and tightening your buttocks. Start with your hands at thigh level, with palms facing out.

2 Inhale as you roll your arms up until your elbows point forwards. Touch your shoulders with the backs of your fingers.

FISH SWIM

This stretch helps to increase circulation to the nerves in the arms and hands. Be sure to keep your palms together and your shoulders relaxed.

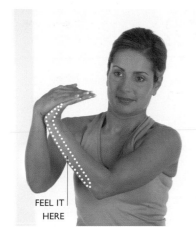

FEEL IT HERE

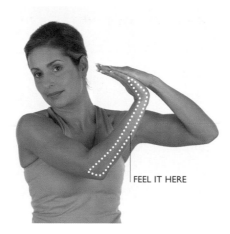

FEEL IT HERE

1 Place your palms together and begin moving your hands as a unit in a horizontal figure-of-eight pattern. Smoothly move your hands down to the left, and then up and around.

2 Continue moving your hands down to the right, and then up and around again. Let your shoulders and head move naturally with the pattern. Repeat 1 times, then reverse direction.

ARM PRESS DOWN

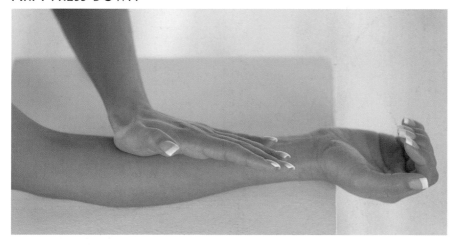

Place your forearm on a firm, flat surface. Place the heel of your other hand on the meaty part of your forearm, just below the elbow, and apply firm pressure. Hold for 4 breath cycles, then repeat on the other arm.

MINI CATALOGUE

Include these additional stretches in your routine. Muscle tightness in the face and upper body also affects the arms and hands.

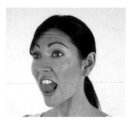

lion stretch p23
say "ahhh" for 5 counts

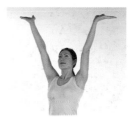

arms open p29
hold for 3 breath cycles

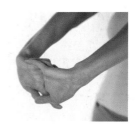

clasped fingers p28
hold for 3 breath cycles

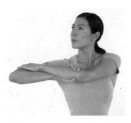

twist, arms crossed p33
hold for 2 breath cycles;
repeat on other side

LOWER BACK

It is estimated that as many as 80 percent of us will experience lower back discomfort at some point in our lives. Try these gentle "relievers" to help ease the pain. Remember to respect your lower back – it takes so much abuse and can truly bring us to our knees if we are not careful.

DIAGONAL KNEE ROCK

Lie down and position a folded towel under your lower back for support. Pressing your lower back into the towel, exhale and slowly bring one knee and then the other to your chest. Generally, the rule is to rock away from the side of the back with discomfort. Hug your knees, and gently rock your knee diagonally towards the opposite shoulder 10 times. Repeat on the other side, if appropriate.

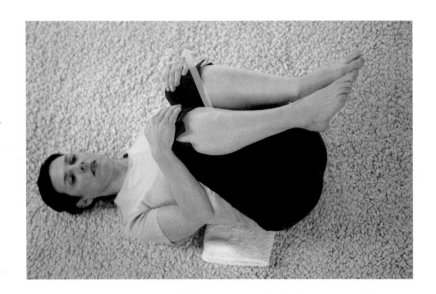

SACRAL CIRCLES

Lie down and position a folded towel under your lower back for support. Pressing your lower back into the towel, exhale and slowly bring one knee and then the other to your chest. Use your hands to circle your knees. Breathe normally as you circle your knees 5 times in each direction.

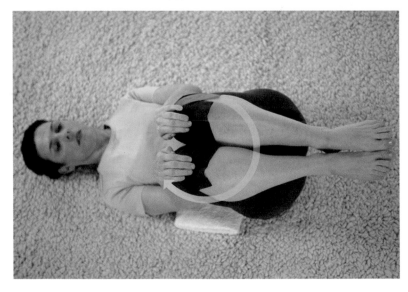

ONE-KNEE HUG

Lie down and position a folded towel under your lower back for support. Bend your knees, keeping both feet on the floor. Press your lower back against the towel, put your hands behind your knee, and gently pull it towards your chest. Stay for 1 breath cycle, then exhale and lower the foot down. Repeat this, alternating legs, 10 times.

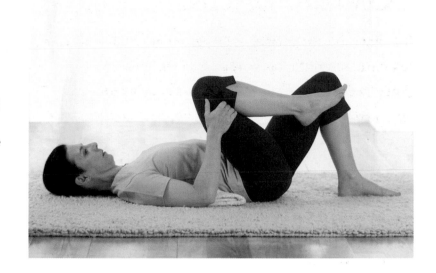

TWO-KNEE HUG

Lie down and position a folded towel under your lower back for support. Bend your knees, keeping both feet on the floor. Press your lower back against the towel and exhale as you lift one thigh then the other and hug your knees to your chest. Stay for 3 breath cycles, then keeping your lower back pressed into the towel, lower one foot then the other. Repeat 2 more times.

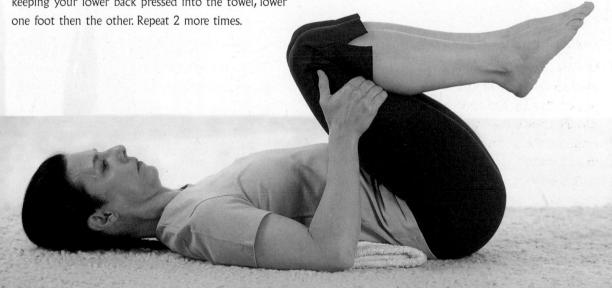

LOW COBRA

Lie on your front. Place your hands, palms down, in front of you and line your elbows up under your shoulders. Press your thighs into the floor and exhale as you hold your abdomen firm and come up on your forearms. Raise your chest, feeling a lengthening in your lower back and abdomen. Hold for 2 breath cycles. Exhale as you lower your chest.

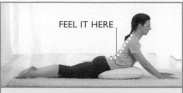

FEEL IT HERE

INTENSIFY THE STRETCH
Position a pillow under your hips and abdomen. Press up higher, lifting your forearms off the floor and pressing into your hands.

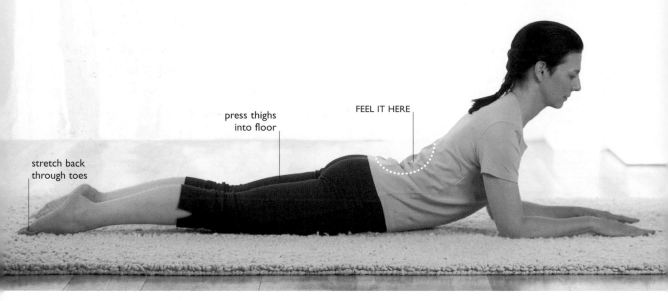

stretch back
through toes

press thighs
into floor

FEEL IT HERE

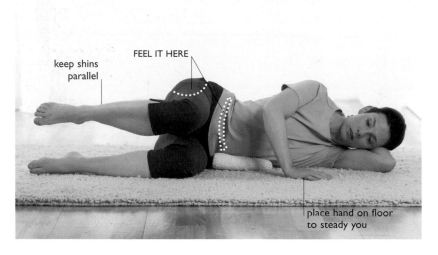

keep shins
parallel

FEEL IT HERE

place hand on floor
to steady you

LYING LEG LIFT

Lie on your side with a folded towel or cushion under your waist. Support your head on your arm. Bend both knees so that they are at a 90° angle to your body. Exhale and unweight your top leg off of your bottom one, keeping your shins parallel. Hold for 1 breath cycle, then slowly lower your leg as you exhale. Do this 5 times, then repeat on the other side.

LYING BACK-RELAXER

Lie on your side with a folded towel or pillow under your waist. Support your head on your arm. Bend your knees slightly, and place a pillow between your legs. Stay in this passive stretch for 4 minutes. Repeat, lying on the other side.

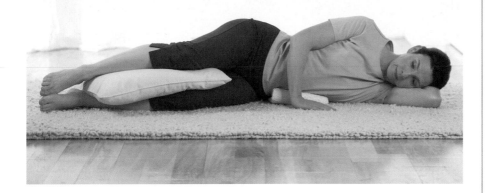

SUPPORTED BACK-RELAXER

Lie on your back, your legs propped up on a chair at 90°. Position a folded towel under your lower back. Exhale and cross your arms over your ribcage so that your hands fall towards the floor. Stay for 2 minutes, and work up to 10 minutes. Focus on breathing regularly.

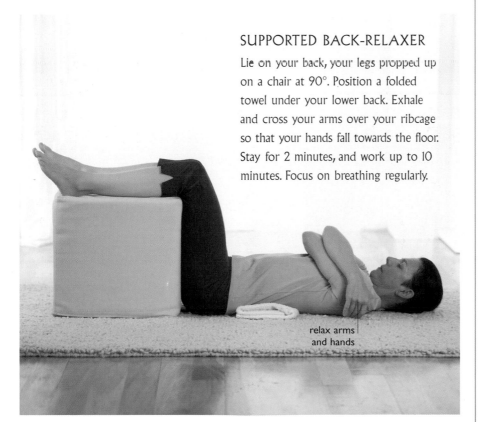

relax arms and hands

MINI CATALOGUE

Stretching your arms, waist, and hips relieves pressure on the spine and will help to keep your back happy.

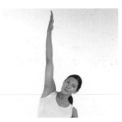

standing side bend *p31*
hold for 4 breath cycles; repeat on other side

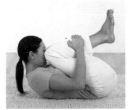

knees to chest *p37*
hold for 2 breath cycles

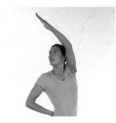

standing waist twist *p40*
hold for 2 breath cycles; repeat on other side

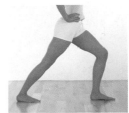

basic lunge *p48*
hold for 4 breath cycles; repeat on other leg

HIPS

Both sitting and standing for long periods can cause discomfort in the hips. They support upper body weight when we are on our feet, and this is intensified by gravity's pull. Add carrying heavy bags or children, and it's little wonder that our hips often feel sore. Try these gentle stretches to help relieve aches and pains.

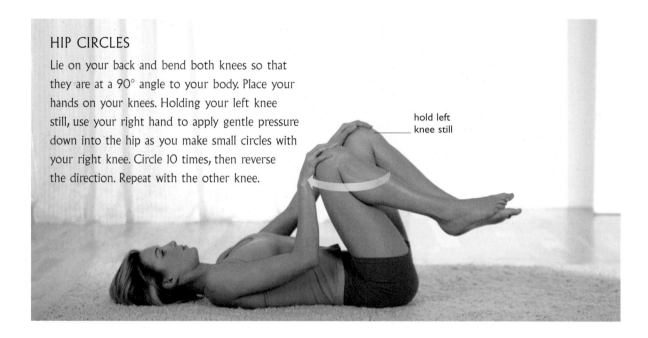

HIP CIRCLES

Lie on your back and bend both knees so that they are at a 90° angle to your body. Place your hands on your knees. Holding your left knee still, use your right hand to apply gentle pressure down into the hip as you make small circles with your right knee. Circle 10 times, then reverse the direction. Repeat with the other knee.

hold left knee still

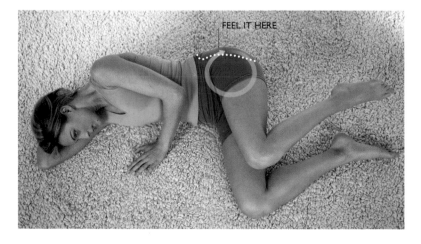

FEEL IT HERE

PELVIC CIRCLES

Lie on your side and support your head on your arm, or a pillow if preferred. Bend both knees so that they are at a 90° angle to your body. Locate the bony bump at the top of your thigh, and use this as an imaginary axis as you form a slow, horizontal circle with your pelvis. Perform 6 circles, then reverse direction. Repeat, lying on your other side.

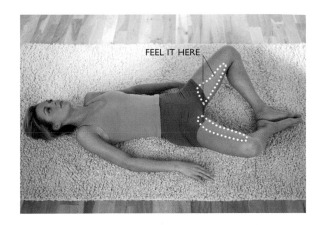

FEEL IT HERE

INVERSE FROG

Lie on your back, and press your lower back firmly into the floor. Place the soles of your feet together, and bend your knees, relaxing them open towards the floor. If your back is pulling off the floor, place a pillow under your pelvis. Stay for 8 breath cycles.

MINI CATALOGUE

These stretches focus on the outer hip muscles and complement the inner hip joint exercises demonstrated on the left.

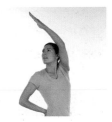

standing waist twist *p40*
hold for 2 breath cycles; repeat on other side

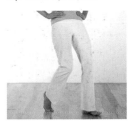

front hip stretch *p42*
hold for 3 breath cycles; repeat on other side

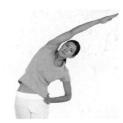

side hip stretch *p43*
hold for 4 breath cycles; repeat on other side

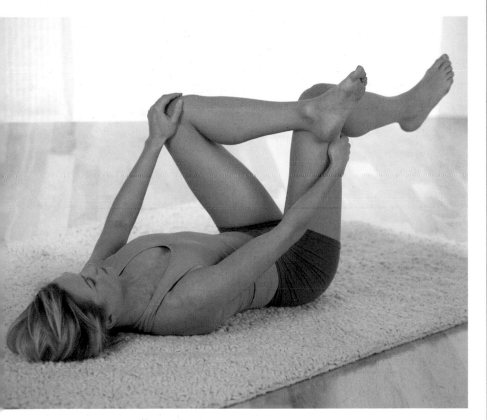

LYING HIP STRETCH

Lie comfortably on the floor. Press your lower back against the floor as you lift one thigh, then the other towards your chest. Cross your left ankle over your right knee. Pull your right thigh as you press your left knee away from you. Feel a good stretch in your left buttock and back of thigh. Hold for 5 breath cycles, then repeat on the other side.

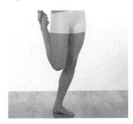

standing quad stretch *p44*
hold for 3 breath cycles; repeat on other side

CALVES

Here are some less obvious lower leg stretches that will affect both the superficial and deep muscles of the calves. Your thoroughness will pay off – tight calves and shins impact the mechanics of the lower back and knees. Go easy with the inner and outer calf and ankle stretches, but apply full pressure on the Calf Ball Press.

CAUTIONS AND TIPS

- **Avoid** the Outer Calf and Ankle Stretch if you have a history of ankle sprains.
- **Do not** perform these stretches for at least four weeks after an ankle sprain.

INNER CALF AND ANKLE STRETCH

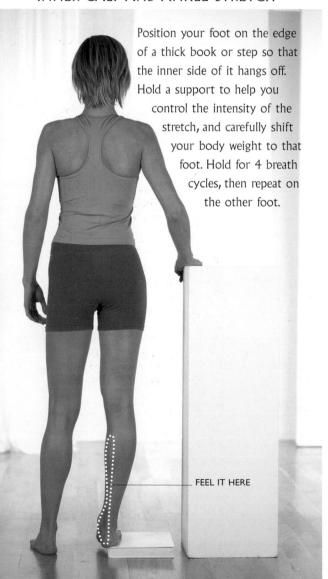

Position your foot on the edge of a thick book or step so that the inner side of it hangs off. Hold a support to help you control the intensity of the stretch, and carefully shift your body weight to that foot. Hold for 4 breath cycles, then repeat on the other foot.

FEEL IT HERE

OUTER CALF AND ANKLE STRETCH

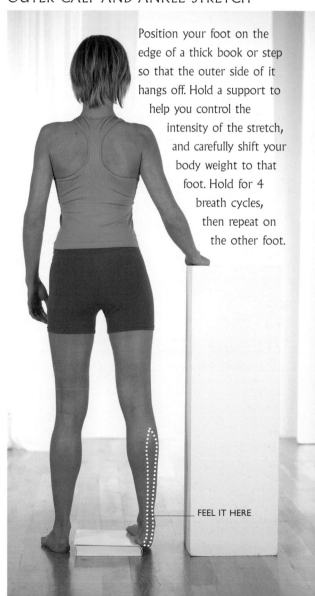

Position your foot on the edge of a thick book or step so that the outer side of it hangs off. Hold a support to help you control the intensity of the stretch, and carefully shift your body weight to that foot. Hold for 4 breath cycles, then repeat on the other foot.

FEEL IT HERE

CALF BALL PRESS

Sit and position a tennis ball under the middle of the meaty part of your calf. Tuck your hips under and lift yourself up with your arms. Place your foot on top of the shin, directly over the tennis ball, and apply pressure for 3 breath cycles. Repeat, targeting tender spots.

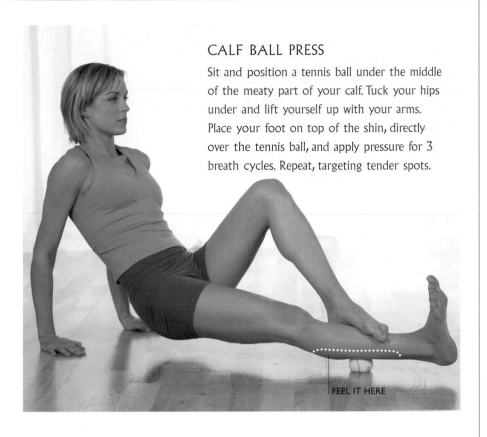

FEEL IT HERE

CALF SHAKE

Sit and raise one leg. Support your thigh with one hand as you shake your calf vigorously with the other. Work up and down the calf, then repeat on the other leg.

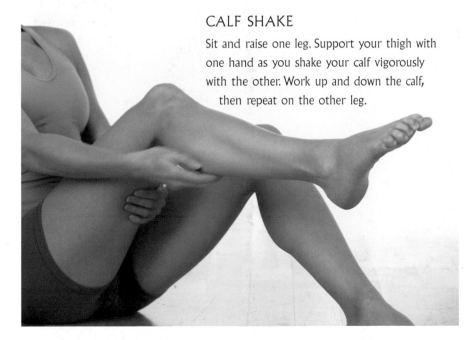

MINI CATALOGUE

Here are more stretches for the calves, but also for the feet and ankles – tightness in these areas can affect the calves.

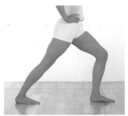

basic lunge *p48*
hold for 4 breath cycles; repeat on other leg

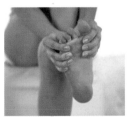

transverse arch *p51*
repeat both steps 5 times on each foot

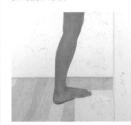

step drop *p49*
hold for 4 breath cycles; repeat on other leg

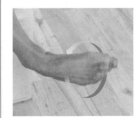

ankle circles *p50*
circle 5 times, each way; repeat on other foot

STRETCHES BY BODY PART

Use this index as a complement to the Head-to-Toe Catalogue of Stretches (*see pp.20–51*) and as a guide to the many other stretches featured in this book. Because a single stretch involves many different muscles, stretches are listed by major body parts and muscle groups, although there is inevitable overlap. In the index opposite, the muscles stretched are listed in bold after each body part. Use the diagrams below to help you locate the different muscles.

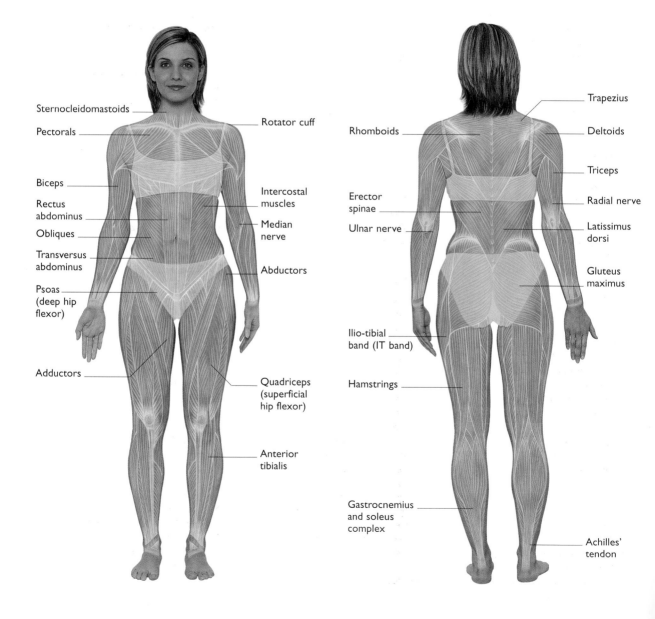

Sternocleidomastoids

Pectorals

Biceps

Rectus abdominus

Obliques

Transversus abdominus

Psoas (deep hip flexor)

Adductors

Rotator cuff

Intercostal muscles

Median nerve

Abductors

Quadriceps (superficial hip flexor)

Anterior tibialis

Rhomboids

Erector spinae

Ulnar nerve

Ilio-tibial band (IT band)

Hamstrings

Gastrocnemius and soleus complex

Trapezius

Deltoids

Triceps

Radial nerve

Latissimus dorsi

Gluteus maximus

Achilles' tendon

HEAD, FACE, EYES

Muscles in the scalp, face, and eyes

Catalogue 22–23
Ear pull 106

NECK

Sternocleidomastoids, Trapezius

Catalogue 24–25
Ear pull 106
Ear-to-shoulder neck stretch 86
Hair pull 22
Hand-on-head neck stretch 97
Hug with head bow 111
Morning wake-up 68–71
Neck and shoulders 140–143
Pendulum head 113

SHOULDERS

Rotator cuff muscles, Deltoids,
Rhomboids, Trapezius, Biceps,
Triceps

Backwards prayer 109
Backwards wrist pull 85
Catalogue 26–27
Curve and arch 88
Elbow grasp 95
Energizing warm-up, st.1–2 76
Hands-behind-back twist 117
Morning wake-up, st.6 70
Pendulums 143
Relaxing wind-down, st.7–11 74–75
Shoulder oval stretch 133
Shoulder rolls 143
Twist punch 111

ARMS AND HANDS

Biceps; Triceps; Ulnar, Median, and Radial
nerves; Latissimus dorsi; forearm and
palm muscles

Arms and hands 144–147
Backwards prayer 109
Catalogue 28–29
Clasped hands back 127
Computer use 104–107
Elbow grasp 95
Elbow stretch 116
Energizing warm-up, st.2, st.12–13
   76–79
Finger splay 137
Leaning triceps stretch 93
Morning wake-up, st.6 70
Pendulums 143
Relaxing wind-down, st.7–11 74–75

Shoulder oval stretch 133
Shoulder rolls 143
Single arm stretch 31
Triceps overhead 83

CHEST AND RIBCAGE

Pectorals, Intercostal muscles

Arc sweep 145
Backwards prayer 109
Backwards wrist pull 85
Ballooning 144
Catalogue 30–31
Chair tilt 104
Chest thrust 136
Crossed arms twist 84
Curve and arch 88
Energizing warm-up, st.2 76
Energizing warm-up, st.6–8 78
Fish 34
Hands-behind-back twist 117
Hips up 35
Low cobra 150
Overhead crossed arms twist 84
Relaxing wind-down, st.7–11 74–75
Seated back twist 113
Seated cobra 106
Seated reach-up 112
Shoulder blade squeeze 120
Standing wind-up 99
Upper back forward stretch 32

UPPER BACK

Erector spinae, Trapezius

Alligator 132
Backwards prayer 109
Ballooning 144
Camel 131
Cat 131
Catalogue 32–35
Chair tilt 104
Clasped hands back 127
Controlled twist 132
Crossed arms twist 84
Cross-legged hang 113
Curve and arch 88
Elbow grasp 95
Energizing warm-up, st.2 76
Energizing warm-up, st.6–8 78
Gentle seated twist 135
Hand-on-head neck stretch 97
Hands-behind-back twist 117
Hug with head bow 111
Low cobra 150

Morning wake-up, st.7–10 70–71
Relaxing wind-down, st.7–11 74–75
Seated back twist 113
Seated cobra 106
Seated spinal roll 134
Shoulder blade squeeze 120
Shoulder oval stretch 133
Shoulder rolls 143
Standing back stretch 109
Standing back twist 123
Standing hand clasp 99
Standing wind-up 99
Twist punch 111
Upper back side-bend and twist 87

LOWER BACK

Latissimus dorsi, Erector spinae

Alligator 132
Ankle-hold hip stretch 94
Ankle reach 135
Ballooning 144
Bowed-head knee hug 96
Camel 131
Cat 131
Catalogue 36–39
Chair tilt 104
Chest thrust 136
Controlled twist 132
Crossed arms twist 84
Crossover leg twist 129
Curve and arch 88
Driver's hamstring stretch 108
Energizing warm-up, st.2 76
Gentle hamstring 130
Gentle seated twist 135
Hands-behind-back twist 117
Hip circles 152
Hip sway 109
Hip tilt 120
Hip walk back 121
Leg unweighting 118
Low cobra 150
Lower back 148–151
Lower back fist press 102
Lying hamstring stretch 128
Lying hip stretch 153
Morning wake-up, st.5 69
Morning wake-up, st.7–10 70–71
Overhead crossed arms twist 84
Pelvic circles 152
Relaxing wind-down, st.7–11 74–75
Seated back twist 113
Seated cobra 106

Seated figure 4 98
Seated piriformis twist 91
Seated reach-up 112
Seated spinal roll 134
Sitting groin stretch 89
Sitting, knees crossed 95
Standing back stretch 109
Standing back twist 123
Standing wind-up 99
Thinker 119
Twist punch 111

WAIST

Rectus abdominus, Transversus abdominis,
Obliques, Erector spinae

Alligator 132
Ankle reach 135
Backwards wrist pull 85
Camel 131
Cat 131
Catalogue 40–41
Chest thrust 136
Controlled twist 132
Crossed arms twist 84
Cross-legged hang 113
Crossover leg twist 129
Energizing warm-up, st.2 76
Energizing warm-up, st.6–8 78
Feet over head 37
Fish 34
Gentle seated twist 135
Hands-behind-back twist 117
Hip sway 109
Hip tilt 120
Hip walk back 121
Hips up 35
Leg-cross hip stretch 43
Lower back 148–151
Lunge with fists in back 122
Lying hip stretch 153
Morning wake-up, st.6–10 70–71
Overhead crossed arms twist 84
Pelvic circles 152
Psoas lunge 92
Relaxing wind-down, st.7–11 74–75
Seated back twist 113
Seated head curl 36
Seated piriformis twist 91
Seated reach-up 112
Seated spinal roll 134
Side hip stretch 43
Standing back stretch 109
Standing back twist 123

Standing wind-up 99
Twist punch 111
Upper back side-bend and twist 87

HIPS AND THIGHS

Psoas, Abductors, Adductors, IT band, Gluteus
maximus, Quadriceps, Hamstrings

Ankle-hold hip stretch 94
Ankle reach 135
Bent-over hip stretch 115
Bowed-head knee hug 96
Catalogue 42–43, 44–47
Cross-legged hang 113
Driver's hamstring stretch 108
Energizing warm-up, st.3–4 77
Gentle seated twist 135
Hands-behind-back twist 117
Hips 152–153
Hip sway 109
Hip tilt 120
Hip walk back 121
Leaning hurdler 89
Leg unweighting 118
Lower back 36–39
Lower back 148–150
Lower back fist press 102
Morning wake-up, st.7–8 70
Pregnancy 128–129
Post pregnancy 130–132
Psoas lunge 92
Relaxing wind-down, st.5–6 73
Relaxing wind-down, st.12 75
Seated figure 4 98
Seated piriformis twist 91
Sitting groin stretch 89
Sitting, knees crossed 95
Standing back stretch 109
Step hip stretch 123
Thinker 119
Walker's lunge 114
Wide squat 126

CALVES AND SHINS

Gastrocnemius and soleus complex, Anterior
tibialis, Achilles' tendon

Ankle circles 50
Ankle reach 135
Calves 154–155
Catalogue 48–49
Cross-legged hang 113
Crossover reach back 39
Feet over head 37
Foot pointer 50

Front hip stretch 42
Front of shin stretch 97
Hanging with crossed arms 38
Hip sway 109
Inner thigh squat 45
Inverse frog 153
Knee circles 103
Leaning hurdler 89
Long walks 114–115
Lunge with fists in back 122
Morning wake-up, st.8 70
Psoas lunge 92
Rolling feet 119
Runner's lunge 90
Side foot stretch 50
Side hip stretch 43
Sitting groin stretch 89
Sitting, knees crossed 95
Standing hamstring 46
Supported hamstring 46
Toe bend 51
Wide squat 126

ANKLES AND FEET

Achilles' tendon; muscles and
tendons in the sole of the foot

Ankle reach 135
Basic lunge 48
Calves 154–155
Catalogue 50–51
Crossover reach back 39
Feet over head 37
Front hip stretch 42
Front of shin stretch 97
Hanging with crossed arms 38
Hip sway 109
Inner thigh squat 45
Long walks 114–115
Knee circles 103
Lunge with fists in back 122
Morning wake-up, st.8 70
Psoas lunge 92
Rolling feet 119
Runner's lunge 90
Side hip stretch 43
Standing hamstring 46
Step drop 49
Supported hamstring 46
Wide squat 126

INDEX

ACKNOWLEDGMENTS

Author's acknowledgments

Thank you to the incredible DK team that made this all possible. It was truly a wonderful experience to work with so many talented people: Nasim Mawji for her fabulous language skills, Miranda Harvey for impeccable design, Russell Sadur for outstanding photography, and Mary-Clare Jerram for fostering the project, as well as the UK office for all their across-the-seas assistance. Especially, I humbly thank my dear beloved husband, for his unyielding loyalty, devotion, and humour.

Publisher's acknowledgments

Dorling Kindersley would like to thank photographer Russell Sadur and his assistant, Nina Duncan, Stephen McIlmoyle for models' hair and make-up, Gunilla Johansson for styling, and the models: Lucy Shakespeare, Gunilla Johansson, Anne Browne, Louise Cole, Sheri Staplehurst, and Zoe Moore. Thanks to Jennifer Williams for her invaluable help. Thanks also to Zoe Moore for editorial assistance, Mark Cavanagh for arrow artworks, Jo Cameron for illustrations, and Claire Cross for proofreading.

ABOUT THE AUTHOR

Suzanne Martin is a doctor of physical therapy with over 25 years' experience in the fields of health and movement. A former dancer, she is a Master trainer certified by the American Council on Exercise. She writes regularly for *Dance Magazine* and *Pilates Style* magazine in the United States, and is well known as an educational presenter within the worlds of Pilates, dance, and physical therapy. Suzanne is the lead physical therapist for the Smuin Ballet in San Francisco and maintains a private practice, Total Body Development, in Alameda, California. For more information, check the website: www.totalbodydevelopment.com.